THE GREATEST WEALTH IN THE WORLD

"The reason for the format of the book is simple. I was tired of seeing too many technical and rather boring plant books on the market. A student who has finished one of them hardly knows the plant at all, and the information is soon forgotten. I believe that each plant has a marvelous story of its own. I have incorporated these stories into the text to add form and dimension to the discussion of each plant. Now the student can know plants intimately, as I do. I want to make the study of plants exciting to the beginner as well as the seasoned herbalist."
— Tom Brown, Jr.

REDISCOVER THE JOYS AND BEAUTY OF NATURE WITH TOM BROWN, JR.

THE TRACKER
Tom Brown's classic true story—the most powerful and magical high-spiritual adventure since *The Teachings of Don Juan*

THE SEARCH
The continuing story of *The Tracker*, exploring the ancient art of the new survival

THE VISION
Tom Brown's profound, personal journey into an ancient mystical experience, the Vision Quest

THE QUEST
The acclaimed outdoorsman shows how we can save our planet

THE JOURNEY
A message of hope and harmony for our earth and our spirits—Tom Brown's vision for healing our world

GRANDFATHER
The incredible true story of a remarkable Native American and his lifelong search for peace and truth in nature

AWAKENING SPIRITS
For the first time, Tom Brown shares the unique meditation exercises used by students of his personal Tracker classes

THE WAY OF THE SCOUT
Tom Brown's newest, most empowering work—a collection of stories illustrating the advanced tracking skills taught to him by Grandfather

AND THE BESTSELLING SERIES OF TOM BROWN'S FIELD GUIDES

Berkley Books by Tom Brown, Jr.

THE TRACKER (as told to William Jon Watkins)
THE SEARCH (with William Owen)
TOM BROWN'S FIELD GUIDE TO
    WILDERNESS SURVIVAL
    (with Brandt Morgan)
TOM BROWN'S FIELD GUIDE TO NATURE
    OBSERVATION AND TRACKING
    (with Brandt Morgan)
TOM BROWN'S FIELD GUIDE TO CITY AND
    SUBURBAN SURVIVAL (with Brandt Morgan)
TOM BROWN'S FIELD GUIDE TO LIVING
    WITH THE EARTH (with Brandt Morgan)
TOM BROWN'S GUIDE TO WILD EDIBLE AND
    MEDICINAL PLANTS
TOM BROWN'S FIELD GUIDE TO THE
    FORGOTTEN WILDERNESS
TOM BROWN'S FIELD GUIDE TO NATURE
    AND SURVIVAL FOR CHILDREN
    (with Judy Brown)
THE VISION
THE QUEST
THE JOURNEY
GRANDFATHER
AWAKENING SPIRITS
THE WAY OF THE SCOUT
THE SCIENCE AND ART OF TRACKING

About the Author

At the age of eight, Tom Brown, Jr., began to learn tracking and hunting from Stalking Wolf, a displaced Apache Indian. Today Brown is an experienced woodsman whose extraordinary skill has saved many lives, including his own. He manages and teaches one of the largest wilderness and survival schools in the U.S. and has instructed many law enforcement agencies and rescue teams.

TOM BROWN'S GUIDE TO WILD EDIBLE AND MEDICINAL PLANTS

Tom Brown, Jr.

Illustrated by Heather Bolyn
and Trip Becker

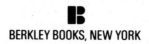

BERKLEY BOOKS, NEW YORK

This Guide contains material, knowledge of which could be invaluable in dealing with a sudden wilderness emergency—an unexpected "survival situation" when knowledge of fundamental survival techniques could be lifesaving. The Guide, however, is *not* a plant identification guide. It is intended to be used in conjunction with other books, to complement plant guides with the Author's own philosophy and stories from personal experience. Nor is the guide intended as a substitute for proper medical care.

Neither the publisher nor the Author claim that techniques in the Guide will cure illness in any situation. Some of the techniques and instructions described in the Guide may be inappropriate for persons suffering from certain physical conditions or handicaps. Misuse of this information could cause serious personal injury for which the Publisher and Author disclaim liability.

I lovingly dedicate this book to my son, Tommy, who during its writing virtually lived without his daddy.

In Memory of Sam Winter, a true child of the wilderness, butchered by a society he did not understand.

CONTENTS

PART THREE

TOM BROWN'S GUIDE TO WILD EDIBLE AND MEDICINAL PLANTS

Introduction

It was in the summer of my twelfth year when Grandfather said that I must learn to hunt like a man. I had to seek out the truths of the real hunt and understand what the hunt was all about, accepting the awesome responsibility and knowing the sacred act the Creator had intended the hunt to be. Certainly, I had killed animals in traps and with throwing sticks but never any big game. Grandfather wanted me to use close-range and primitive hunting techniques to bring me nearer to the actual kill. Previous to this, hunting had been matter-of-fact, with only token thought, prayer, and appreciation given to the killing of the animal. We were young and not very experienced in survival and the laws of Creation. We meant no disrespect, we just did not know any better, and our prayers and appreciation were mere imitations of Stalking Wolf's devotion. There was no awe or intensity of feelings, we were mere babes in the woods, connected to, yet still removed from the soil. We didn't feel the reality of the umbilical cord connecting us and Earth Mother.

Grandfather's ambition was to show me the reality of the hunt, of killing and dying, and of appreciation and sacrifice through the only way it could be truly learned—by doing it. The rules were simple enough. Within one week I was to locate a small deer, track it, stalk it, and take its life, using a stone knife lashed to a short stick. Traps had been so very easy: I had only to set and bait the trap, then walk away and do something else for the rest of the day while the trap did the rest. I was totally removed from the *act* of killing. The trap provided a supermarket-type effect where the animal was already dead and near ready to cook. The close-range hunt took all of my skills, so much patience, and a tremendous amount of time to complete. It was the real hunt, lost to the hunters of today.

Modern hunters kill from long distances. They sit waiting in tree stands or blinds, use binoculars, scopes, and so many other modern devices, all designed to remove the hunter from the actual killing. I strongly doubt if many of today's hunters can track their game, stalk within a few feet, and finally kill it. Their long-range arrows with compound bows and their high-power rifles make the task of killing easy. Modern hunters lack the basic and ancient skills, and thus lack the understanding of what the true hunt and hunter is all about. Grandfather did not want me to fall into this same complacency.

I began my hunt with many hours of deep thought and introspection, spending time alone to try and put things into perspective. I fasted for four days so that I could understand hunger and appreciate the gift of food the deer would provide. I took sweatlodge to purify myself and asked the Creator to help me with the hunt. Without the Creator's approval, there would be no hunt and no game. Grandfather helped me through all these things so that I would fully understand the sacred act I was about to perform. It was important to make the hunt right in my mind so that I would prove worthy of the gift of life I was about to receive. I had to realize that I was a predator and a very intricate part of Creation. I had to recapture my birthright.

I left the camp in the early morning, armed with a flint knife. I wandered miles away from camp, relying on my inner feelings to guide me to the proper hunting area. I kept careful watch on the tracks and the landscape, looking for signs of a crippled or sick deer. I had to follow the laws of the predators, and could not take a healthy animal. Predators kill only those animals that are too sick or weak to survive, thus contributing to the continuation of the herd. I did not want to break that sacred tradition. Finally, my eyes caught the tracks of a small yearling deer with a defect in his right rear leg. He couldn't have weighed over forty-five pounds and I was sure that he could never make it through the summer, far less through the winter. Choosing him as my deer, my gift of life, I prayed that the kill would be quick.

I tracked him for hours. His tracks followed his mother's, but showed much trouble negotiating the tougher areas of the landscape. He tired easily and spent much of his time resting or trying to catch up to his mother. The more I studied the tracks, the more I understood this little deer. His bad leg was not a result of a recent injury but either some kind of birth defect or an injury that occurred around the time of his birth. After a full day of tracking, it was painfully apparent to me that he could not run, but hobbled away feebly at the approach of danger. My heart went out to this little deer, so desperately hanging onto life, and I grew sick with the thought of what I had to do.

For several days I watched the little deer. I became very familiar, almost intimate, with his travels and routines. I tracked him, watched him, slept near him and his mother, knew where he fed, drank, and played. Strangely, I felt part of the little group and was so close, as a matter of fact, that they stopped paying attention to me. Certainly, at first, they were very skittish, but as the days progressed, they saw me as no threat. I became as natural as anything on the landscape, a very deadly mistake for any deer, even a healthy one. Many times I got within only a few feet of the little one, once even close enough to touch him. So many times I could have killed him, but I wanted a clean kill and Grandfather had said that he wanted me to know my animal intimately.

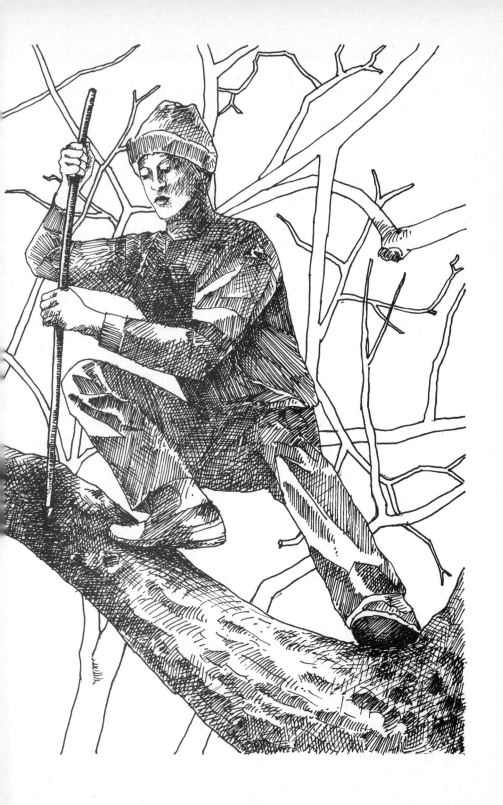

I began to look at the whole affair as a predator, especially when the novelty of the close encounters became commonplace. A huge chess game began to play in my head, with me against the little deer, luring him into a perfect position and situation to give me an advantage and a clean kill. I watched every move and every look. I knew so much about the deer's movements, even better than they did. Their routine would be the cause and the end of the little deer's life. That same deadly routine became ingrained in complaisancy; moving so often the same way, they forgot to be aware. A routine that turns into a life-threatening rut happens not only to deer, but to humans as well. I realized that if I ever allowed myself into a rut it would be certain death, just like it was going to be for the little deer.

My thought patterns became abstract, concentrating only on the hunt—the chess game. The life of the deer became the furthest thing from my mind, and the whole hunt lacked any visible emotion. It was as if I were outside the whole situation looking in, watching the hunter come closer and closer to the final act. My hunger was intense, my body tired, and I knew that the final moves had to be taken. I knew of a tree near a distant field where the little deer stood momentarily every day before he crossed the field. The concentration on the field and the heavy cover of the little tree would distract the deer enough for me to make a move without being noticed beforehand.

The thrill of the oncoming hunt overpowered all other thoughts and emotions. I strapped my flint knife onto a long, thin stick and took a few flakes from the flint to make it deadly sharp. My moves had been planned and replanned until my head was swimming with the mental practice. I would sit in the tree just before the time of the day when the little deer's routine would bring him to the edge of the field. When he got into his usual position, I would drop from the tree and drive my spear through his back and between his shoulder blades, using the momentum of my jump to drive the spear deep. If he didn't die immediately, I would then track him to the point where he died.

I was in the tree, concealed and waiting, an hour before the little deer usually came to the field. I had darkened and camouflaged my body with mud and natural herbs. My internal dialogue was shut down with a constant prayer and concentration on the hunt. Every leaf seemed to speak, not a sound or movement on the landscape went unnoticed: Everything had something important to do with the hunt and could not be overlooked. Every creature, every plant, the weather, wind, and earth were all players in this eternal game of death, of life giving to life. I had to be aware on all levels, physically and emotionally. I had to surpass all thought and allow my instincts and reactions to take over completely.

The deer approached the field right on time, his mother was up wind and a few hundred feet down field. As he had done hundreds of times before, he walked under the tree and stopped to survey the open field. There was no fear in him because nothing in his routine was broken, nothing on the landscape was out of place. With no thoughts in my head, allowing the predator within to take over, I dropped from the upper branches of the tree, onto his small back. I thrust the spear through one side of the deer's back, off my intended mark by a few inches, but he went down. He thrashed, crippled in the hind legs because part of the spinal column had been severed, but still alive. In a fit of rage at my own failure at a clean kill, and fired by the awesome instincts of the predator, I began to choke the little deer to death.

It seemed to take hours to kill him. I was half out of my mind with the power of the kill when suddenly my eyes caught the eyes of the deer as he slowly died. A shock came over me as I now regained human consciousness, coming slowly to my senses. I gazed into the terror in his eyes, my hands trembling as I cut off his breath, my mind racing back to the week before and the way I knew this little deer as a brother. Another shudder from the deer brought me back to his eyes, but this time the terror was replaced by understanding and release. In that moment of intense eye contact, the deer knew that he was to become my life's blood; there was no struggle, only a knowing acceptance.

I fell off of him, exhausted. My body shook, not with excitement for the hunt, but with tears. His blood covered me and mixed with my sweat. I grew nauseous at the thought of what I had done. Natural order of things or not, I felt sick and disgusted with the whole killing. I knew this little deer as a brother, I followed him, watched him feed, and slept close to him for many nights. Now it was over. I had removed this deer from the flow of life, and I felt no better than a murderer. I just could not make sense of it all, nor could I ever forgive myself for this vicious act, sacred or not.

Still sobbing, I threw his body over my shoulders and headed back to camp. He was so light and sickly that I could hardly feel his weight. Except for the warm blood that ran down my chest and back, his presence was almost imperceptible. Thoughts raced through my head as I tried to justify his death. Certainly, I needed the meat to survive, and his flesh would find a rebirth in my flesh; but why did it have to be that way? Why the pain? Why couldn't we eat plants instead of inflicting pain on another animal?

I knew killing now. It wasn't easy and removed, like pulling back a bow or the trigger of a gun, allowing the arrow or bullet to do the killing. I felt the pain and loss known only to those who have felt an animal's spirit slip through their fingers. I knew the awesome responsibility of the sacred hunt and the ultimate sacrifice of life giving to life. I would never kill again without feeling this pain and sacrifice. My prayers to the hunt would never be parroted emptily or without conviction. I knew the hunt.

The trip seemed endless, the demons of my mind swirled like clouds. So many questions unanswered, so much guilt, so many crushing and debilitating emotions. I tried desperately to make sense of it all. The tears and sobs were endless. My heart felt as if it were ripped from my chest, and there was no way out of my pain and sorrow. I had lost a friend, a brother, and couldn't really justify his death. Would it not have been in the natural order of things to let him die of starvation this winter? Why do we have to be the caretakers, and how can I be part of this sacred cycle if I felt so much pain? In my mind I was denying that humankind was a necessary and intricate part of things, regardless of what Grandfather was trying to show us to the contrary.

As I walked up the path to camp, I caught sight of Grandfather leaning against a tree, watching me. In a way I hated him for making me kill in this way. As I drew closer, I made no attempt to hide my tears but gazed right into his eyes. For a fleeting moment, I caught the same glimmer the deer had in his eyes, the all-knowing feeling. He plainly saw my pain and suffering. He sensed the myriads of questions flowing through my mind, as I know now he must have had at one time. He pointed an old and gnarled finger at me and said, "Grandson, when you can feel the same pain and suffering for a blade of grass ripped from the Earth as you do for that deer, you will truly be one with all things."

His words hit me like a hammer. The death of rabbits in my traps and the plants and trees torn from the ground to feed me had given me no pain in the past because I was removed from the killing. Now I understood fully. To be appreciated and respected, a thing need not be living, breathing, and warm-blooded, or have eyes and be considered cute; everything is composed of the same spirit that moves through all things, and all equally sacrifice their lives for our lives. The only difference is that up to this time I could not feel the pain of the plants, I could not hear them scream or see them bleed. It wasn't that we should give up killing deer or animals because they are like us, but that we should realize we are part of the spirit that moves through all things. Everything is equal if we listen with our hearts and not our minds.

Ever since his words were spoken, I have been on a quest to find the oneness of which Grandfather spoke. Over the years, I have found that oneness. I have learned to feel the pain and hear the voices of all living things. I know that all things are equal and should not be judged on some manmade merit system or evolutionary ladder. Beyond that, I have learned that everything is composed of that spirit: water, earth, sky, and wind. They all contribute to life, every part a piece of an overall puzzle, everything necessary to the whole. When something is needlessly killed or removed from the flow of life with no forethought or feeling, then it is part of all things that are dying. We move within the realm of Creation, and Creation moves in us; there is no inner or outer dimension. Our quest should be to break down the walls and learn to be one with all things. This book, then, becomes your doorway.

PART ONE

The Gardener Attitude

Many people think that survivalists and herbalists are not unlike a swarm of locusts swooping down on the landscape and devouring everything. This can't be further from the truth. A good survivalist and herbalist actually can do more good for any landscape than a person that does nothing at all. The area where I hold all of my advanced classes is a good working example of the principle I call the gardener or caretaker attitude. We have been using that area of the Pine Barrens for six years, running eight classes a year with thirty-five students in each class. We support all the class activities on one section of forest, about thirty acres in all. Ironically, this area has become a Garden of Eden, in balance in the way the old Pinelands used to be. It has become a mecca for animals during the winter season when their home territory runs out of food. Compared to other areas of the Pinelands it is the best in every way, a place of harmony for the Creator's creatures.

The reason for this change is simple: We have entered this area with an attitude of caretaker. Seeing the imbalance and feeling the responsibility toward these brothers and sisters thwarted in their encroaching development, we lovingly cared for them. The stream was opened up in one place, overgrowth harvested from another. We sensed what healing was necessary and cared for our little area. The results speak for themselves. For generations, we have been a society of people who have killed their grandchildren to feed their children. Our approach to nature is that it is here for us to use or abuse at our own discretion. We never had to answer to anyone for the rape of the land because we felt that we owned the land, whether by virtue of our position on the evolutionary ladder or by decree from the Creator. Well the time of judgment is at hand and we will have to pay for what we have done. Every landscape in this nation is out of balance and someone has to yell "stop!"

We can no longer take from the land thoughtlessly. We must look into the future to see what effects our actions will have on our grandchildren and their children's children, and we must begin to do something now to get the land back into balance. It is going to take drastic measures, each person doing what they can to make things right again. If we believe in the old saying that we are the caretakers

9

of the Earth, we should be ashamed of the way we have taken care of it. We now have to become new caretakers with much forethought, prayer, and dedication to doing things right. We have to pay for and set straight the mistakes of our forefathers, or there will be nothing left to sustain life.

Anytime we enter the landscape, we should look at it as a gardener looks at his garden, or as a caretaker oversees his grounds. Then we should weed, trim, and propagate the land to get it back into balance and harmony. We have been given a sacred duty to help bring back the Earth to what it once was. No, we can't do away with all civilization—I am not an advocate of that change—but we can strike a balance between the modern world and the ancient. The ancient philosophies are as real today as they were yesterday, and if we can integrate the Earth Mother philosophy into our modern one, thereby taking care of what we have left, then this planet can become an utter utopia.

Survival, and the ultimate use of our plant brothers as food and healers, becomes a doorway to the past. We can regain the Earth connection. Any developer or land slayer who has lived totally from the Earth, re-establishing the umbilical connection, could no more destroy the Earth than he could kill his mother. The old ways and the caretaker attitude should never be allowed to die, for if they die, it will not be long before we do, too.

There is such a difference in the caretaker attitude versus the rapist attitude. With the latter, for example, if a man were looking for a bowstave, he would go out to the landscape and search out a stave that was in easy reach. There would be little forethought or care involved in taking the bow, nor would the surrounding landscape be taken into consideration. Typically he would take from the edge of a field a small tree growing straight and tall. It would be virtually knot-free and, to the untrained eye, a very easy bow to work. Unfortunately, the end results of this kind of butchering are poor. Not only does the removal of the tree from the edge of the field prove detrimental to the ecosystem, taking away potential food and cover for the animals, but that kind of bowstave makes a very poor bow. The little sapling has never had to fight, the growth rings are spaced evenly and wide, thus producing a bow that is substandard in cast and snap. Removing a healthy tree from the land does no good at all for the tree, for the overall landscape, or for the person's purposes.

The ancient Native American would remove a bowstave far differently then the rapist. His was the unselfish way, making sure that the land was better for his children and his grandchildren. He understood his position in the overall scheme of things, seeing the oneness, the spirit that moves through all things. Realizing his connection to the Earth, he could not destroy it in any way, for the Earth was truly his Mother. And so, everything that grew from the Earth was of the same blood, brothers and sisters whom he respected dearly. There was no superiority; in fact, often they were not only his food and tools but his teachers. With all these things understood, he would pray for the bowstave, because the awesome responsibility of taking life was a cherished gift. Everything had to be thought out and planned with the utmost care. The future of his people was riding on his decision.

He would be guided out onto the landscape more by feeling than from thought. He may have to search for days and travel many miles before he found the proper stave. In all cases, the land and its needs were always considered before his. Finally, there would be a grove of small saplings that would catch his eye. It would be a grove whose trees were in constant battle with each other. Saplings rubbing up against each other, some dying, many dead. He would approach the grove and make prayers and offerings, telling the trees what he needed, asking permission. The man and the trees understood each other because they spoke a common tongue, the language of the heart. A small sapling was selected and, after the proper prayers, cut down. This ritual was necessary. It showed that in the act of killing a living, growing thing, it was removed from the flow of life to give him life.

The sapling was usually dead or near dying. It was one that fought all its life then gave up. It would make a fine bow because the growth rings were tight and compact, holding a tremendous power born of its fight in life. He would not stop there because he was the caretaker of the Earth and his sacred duty must be completed. He would weed out some of the dead trees, giving the others relief, but leaving other potential bows for people yet to come. Always he would think of the future of his people, especially the children. His was the duty to propagate and care for the land, and thus propagate and care for his children and his grandchildren.

The bowstave was then worked carefully and methodically. Not only was it a gift of life from the tree, but a gift from the Creator. A sloppy job would only bring the wrath of the Creator upon him and his people. He would show the Great Mystery how he felt about the gift by treating it with respect and showing what a good job he could do. Deeper understandings would be gained as the bow was being shaped. From the death of the little tree comes more death, the death of animals. Yet in all this death there is life for his people. The bow becomes an extension of the arm, the flesh is reborn in his flesh. He can then go forth and care for the land so that more bow people and animals will have homes, caring for their futures also.

Many people feel that this attitude toward the landscape, where we decide what is to live and what is to die, is much like playing God. Maybe so, but someone has to do it before it is too late. For all too long we have paid no heed to the land or the flow of life. We do not have the luxury of allowing nature to take its course because we are too late for that. We have to step in now before it is impossible to do anything about it and too late to reverse the poisoning process.

If we adopt this attitude toward the plants and their use, we can only affect the land in a positive way. Whenever we enter the landscape to reap the food and medicines of edible plants, to practice survival living, or for any other purpose, we should be constantly aware of our sacred duties. We are the protectors and caretakers of this planet and must do what is necessary to get things back in balance. However, if you are not sure what to do or how to improve the land, then leave it alone. This knowledge cannot be learned in books or schools. It can be only learned by experience and listening to the voices of Creation, heard only by the heart.

Communication with Nature

Before any real communication with the entities of the Earth begins, we must realize that we are not superior to nature, but an equal part of it all. This acknowledgment of connection must not be a cortical assumption, but assimilated into the very marrow of our existence. Establishing the Earth connection and the unity of self with the entities of the Earth in a balanced equality is the primal step in dynamic communication with Creation and the Creator. This was one of the first and most important lessons I learned. It helped me transcend the purely physical approach to nature, thus opening the spiritual world.

For the first few years of my apprenticeship with Grandfather, I held a rather superior and arrogant attitude toward nature. The better my survival skills and techniques became, the more distant I grew from the natural world. I felt very much as the white man did when he first came to this country, as if nature were there for my use and I could do as I wished. I did have a healthy respect for the storms and potential hazards of the natural world, but at times I looked down on dumb Creation as if it were beneath my dignity even to consider its existence. I felt aloof and removed from the Earth, never realizing that this attitude was standing in the way of my ever becoming one with Creation. Grandfather quickly shook me of my stupid notion by teaching me a very viable lesson—the lesson of reality.

It was late January and we were camped on a small bluff overlooking a snowy field. The night was calm and clear but bitter cold, a penetrating, deep, damp cold for which the Pine Barrens are famous. We had built a warm shelter, our traps had been successful, and we were well fed. A warm fire crackled, throwing its glowing warmth deep into the night, and I felt triumphant and at peace with myself and the way this survival outing was going. I gazed out upon the snow field and saw a young gray fox hunting at its distant end. In the moonlight, he looked as though he had been dipped in liquid silver, and the whole scene seemed frozen in the bitter cold. I felt sorry for the fox and said that I was sure he envied our warm fire and shelter.

I thought that Grandfather had been sleeping, but the statement about the fox snapped him awake. The usual peaceful expression in his eyes was replaced by a definite anger. He smiled, though, and said, "Do not look down upon that which is your teacher and your better. If you do, you will never learn the secrets of Creation." I argued with Grandfather, more out of embarrassment for incurring his wrath than in defense of the casual but ignorant statement I had

13

made. I defended myself by saying that the fox looked cold and hungry, had no sense of reason, and could not make tools or fine shelters. He would be more content lying by our fire and feasting on our leftover rabbits. Grandfather simply stated that the fox needed no tools, shelters, or warm fires, for he was the ultimate survival tool, unlike us humans who could not even go away from our fire without being fully dressed and cut off from Creation. The fox was part of the flow of life, a perfect blend of spirit to Earth; we were the aliens because we were so removed and could not go very far without our tools. We argued until late, never resolving anything. I went to sleep rather angry and upset that no one could see things my way.

I awoke early in the morning to new snow. It was much colder than it had been all week. I reached for my capote, but it was gone. Worried now, I looked for my bow drill and knife to start a fire, but they were gone also. I started to panic, but figured that Grandfather or Rick had borrowed them to make a fire and were probably outside waiting for me. As I looked out the door, my heart fell to my feet, for in the place of last night's fire was a huge snow drift, and there was no sign of Grandfather or Rick. My body shaking with cold and my mind swirling in panic, I dug into the snow to find a rock to make a bow drill, but only succeeded in freezing my hands. Hoping to find a small chip of gravel, I worked my way to the river, but with no luck since the river banks were frozen solid. Upon returning to my shelter, I found that it had collapsed from the addition of last night's snow, which I had failed to clean off in my complacency.

I became angry and irrational, panic overtaking my mind and body, making me feel alien and helpless. I had no choice but to try to walk to my home, many miles away. The only fires burning within me were my anger at Grandfather and Rick for playing such a stupid trick on me, and the realization that I had failed in a rather simple survival situation. I never saw that Grandfather was trying to teach me something very valuable. By taking away all my tools and supplies, he had rendered me helpless and knocked my ego down quite a few pegs, but I never comprehended this lesson until the very end.

I had walked miles and my body ached. The cold had intensified along with the wind, and I shivered violently. I began to run as the terror of freezing to death became a reality. I don't know how far I ran, or even in what direction, before I finally collapsed. I found myself face down in the snow, feeling as if I wanted to go to sleep. I knew hypothermia very well and knew that I was about to die, but there was no fight left in me to do anything to save myself. I looked up out of the snow for what I thought would be the last time when

I saw the fox again, this time standing just a few feet from me. I don't know if it was real or imagined, but I could have sworn he was laughing at me as he trotted off, part of the natural world, needing nothing but himself. At once, I admired the fox and wished that I were he, unencumbered by tools, skills, or supplies, never needing a fire or shelter. I realized what a fool I had been not to seek the fox out as a teacher or, for that matter, to examine closely any of the other things I had taken for granted for so long.

I awoke in Grandfather's shelter, no longer angry but glad to be alive. I felt that a doorway had opened up to me, a doorway that, once passed through, would enrich forever my life. Stalking Wolf was not my only teacher now; I had a forest full of them. I saw new worlds open up to me, and I saw a dynamic way of learning that would bring me closer to a fuller understanding of our Earth Mother, closer to the oneness that I was so desperately seeking. Armed with this new knowledge, I no longer felt alone or aloof but now walked with so many brothers and sisters, forever part of the spirit that moves through all things. I finally realized during the moments when I was near death that all life is equal. It makes no difference what man considers alive or dead, for everything has a spirit and should be respected as an equal.

The Sacred Approach

Communication with the plant and animal people begins with the realization that we are not superior but equal to the plants and animals. In fact, we should begin to understand that in most cases we rank below them in our basic ability to survive. We must learn to use them as teachers and professors in nature's university and to recognize them as providing the best, most viable path to learning anything of the natural ways. The easiest way to begin is to follow many of the simple customs, traditions, and ceremonies used by the ancients from the dawn of time. In these simple services, you will find the basis of all understanding and communication and a way of making sense out of your place in the natural world.

My process of communication begins long before I enter the natural world to take a life. Whether it is plant or animal, even rock, water, or soil, I follow these few basic principles when removing a life from the Earth. First, I must put the act of taking a life into perspective by establishing an extreme need for the act. This perspective is achieved through deep thought about the life and my needs, through introspection, and through much prayer. Thought helps me define my needs, put the act into a clearer perspective, and establish definitely that I need something and that there is no waste. Introspection helps me define my place in the overall scheme of things so that I do not feel superior, and it assures me that the life I will take from the natural world is not taken in profane or mindless manner. I must understand the sacred responsibility given to me by the Creator. Prayer serves not only to communicate with the life I am about to take, but also to communicate with the Creator so that the act is done in a sacred manner. All this reflection lays the foundation for basic communication with that entity and with the voices of the Earth as well.

After the need is established and the taking of a life justified, I go out and begin to wander over the landscape, and I wait for the gift of life to reveal itself to me. Following my heart and not my mind, I look carefully for just the right life. The heart is where all the communication occurs, and it knows exactly what life to take, how to take it, and when. At the time that the animal, plant, or inanimate object reveals itself, I sit by it for a while. Talking to it and praying to the Creator, I ask that my actions be blessed and make a promise

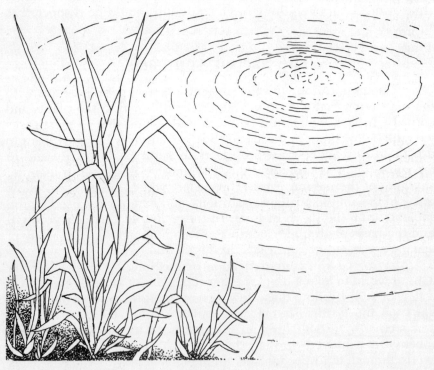

to perpetuate its people. Everything must feel right, or I will move on to another place and other prospects.

Once the life I am looking for is established, I make an offering of sacred tobacco as a token of my appreciation for the life. I can make this offering to the plant itself, another plant nearby, or the Creator. It makes no difference where I place the offering, for the Creator is in all things and all are connected. It is this act of appreciation that causes the whole thing to make sense. It is a gift of life through death, a gift of infinite understanding and deep communication. I then remove that entity from the flow of life with the utmost reverence, and carry it back to camp as I would a fallen brother or warrior. Nothing is wasted or destroyed senselessly. All is in balance.

The act of utilizing this animal or plant is just a continuation of the reverence for life established during the whole process of collection. Everything is done carefully and lovingly. Nothing negative should be found within the feelings of the maker, as the object he is working on will pick up that emotion. The maker should always show care and reverence for fear that the spirit of the plant or animal or, worse yet, the Creator will be offended. It is important that we have the utmost respect for all the gifts given to us by the Creator. After all, all things come from him and through him. I feel that if improper reverence is shown, it will create bad medicine and make things even more difficult. Ultimately, the life should become an extension of yourself, a part of you forever.

Toward a Deeper Communication

Once the feeling of equality with Creation is assimilated into the very essence of your being, and the reverence for all spirits becomes a reality, then the doorway to a deeper communication with the Earth opens. At first, the communication and connection comes to a person almost imperceptibly. It may begin as a gut feeling or a certain subconscious knowledge, eventually taking form as a basic language that we can understand. We find that Nature and Creation do not speak the tongue of man, they speak the universal language of the heart. Many years may pass between the first nuances of communication and true dynamic understanding, but all along the way there are tremendous physical and spiritual rewards. Each brings us closer to a deeper understanding of self and our connection to the Earth Mother.

The best way to start communicating with the plant and animal world is simply to talk to it. For years now, many people have been talking to their houseplants or gardens with tremendous results. It has been shown that the reactions of plants can be registered on sophisticated polygraphs. Even though communications with the plant world go far beyond science, at least in the broadest sense, plants do react. The more you talk to plants, the more you will understand them on deeper levels. Forget about trying to make sense out of the conversation or justify it on a logical level, because it just won't work. Accept that your voice and your attempt to communicate with the plants are real, and you will understand far beyond common thought.

Look also to the plants, animals, rocks, waters, winds, and soils as teachers. At first, these entities do not teach in a classical sense but on deeper levels. You will learn a great deal about the natural world by just observing and trying to understand how the plants or animals fit into the overall scheme. You will soon discover that these entities have the same mother—Earth Mother—who is our mother also. This makes us brothers and sisters to all of Creation. As mentioned previously, all the entities of Creation are professors in nature's university, if we can only figure out how to learn from them. Keen observation and keen awareness will lead you down the path to deeper understanding.

Beyond the basic communication level of talking to and learning from plants, there lies another level of language. This language is derived from our basic instinct, which is at the center of our communication and understanding of the natural world. Each of us is connected to an ancient past and is subject to the same laws that govern all of Creation. The Creator gave each of its creatures certain instincts that keep him alive and are basic to his survival. Mankind still possesses these basic instincts of survival and connection, but they are now overshadowed by his logical thinking. Logic stands in the way of our awareness of the natural world and of the myriad voices that speak to us every day.

Logic and man's ability to solve problems are basic tools that have kept the human race alive for countless years. However, logic is so much a part of our existence today that it virtually rules our mind, body, and emotions. What man needs today, if he is to understand fully the natural world and his place in it, is a blend of logic and instinct. Another name for instinct is intuition, and we rely on this intuition so little that it is almost nonexistent. Our intuition is a key to success in communication, if we could only learn to tap and utilize it.

Getting in touch with our basic instincts or intuition is quite easy at first, if we are willing to let go of logic. The drive for explanations of things is one of the walls that stands in the way of using our intuitions. Sometimes we just have to go with feeling, for feeling is the way we interpret instinct. Instinct and intuition hit us on a purely emotional level, and it is this true emotional level that we must learn to interpret and utilize in all areas of our existence, not only in the natural world. If we would only learn to stop and ask ourselves "How does this feel?" we would begin to tap this tremendous resource of emotion-transmitted instinct.

At first, we begin to feel things about the natural world on an emotional level. We begin to know instinctively something about a plant, animal, or survival situation, and we are not sure how we know. All of us have had the feeling that we were being watched when there was no logical or physical explanation for the feeling, only to find out later that we were being watched. This is only one of myriad intuitions and instincts that we can tap. Intuition and instinct let us know what a plant is good for and whether it is edible or not. Do you think that a doe takes her fawn out and shows her each of the plants she can and cannot eat? Is a dog taught which plants can be eaten to help his digestion? Absolutely not, for all things edible and medicinal are known to animals instinctively. The same instincts run true in mankind also, for the Creator gives all Creation the same gifts. Man's only problem is that his logic interferes with and distorts his basic, primal instincts.

We must learn to get back in touch with these instincts so that they will lead us to a deeper understanding of plants. I do caution you, however, that you must never rely on instinct alone to determine whether a plant is edible or medicinal, for the logical mind can play tricks and is too bound up in emotions. We can at least tap it to understand plants more deeply, as the ancients once did. It was not uncommon to hear Native Americans say, "If you want to know what a plant is good for, then just ask it." They are a people of the Earth, living life close to the Mothering power, relying more on their instincts, intuitions, and spirituality than an overworked logic, thus blending in perfect harmony with the land. Communication on an instinctual level is as common to them as reading a book is to us.

So it is these instincts and intuitions that will add a deeper meaning to our relationship with the Earth. Asking ourselves how we feel about something or sensing a certain communication will give us answers to some very complex questions. But how can we learn to use these instincts and feelings in a more definite, living manner? How can we learn to go beyond logic into the realm of emotion-transmitted instincts and intuitions? How can we make our gut feeling about something become a reality as commonly as we use our logic? Is there any way to improve our communication with our deeper selves, and thus improve our communication with the universe? Fortunately, there is a way to teach people to rely more on their instincts and tap that resource with certainty.

Getting in Touch with Instinct

There is a very easy and basic way of getting in touch with our gut feelings, instincts, or intuitions. Though this method cannot be proven, its results will be very profound and will easily make a believer out of anyone. The necessity of getting in touch with our instincts and intuitions is paramount in learning to communicate with the natural world. This exercise takes a rather vague area of our lives and makes it concrete and usable. It is the best way I know of to reach a vast wellspring of inner resources that will guide us through the natural world with a new, refreshing outlook and will bring us closer to the oneness that we all so desperately seek. First, we must examine the vast power and resources of the mind and the way it makes our connection to the Earth a reality.

The power of the mind is nothing less than incredible. The mind literally sorts out an innumerable amount of information every second, analyzes it, then returns it to our consciousness for evaluation. We are all alert creatures, being struck with stimuli every moment. Our mind automatically sorts out these bits of information and gives us only what is important to us. Much of the information must be tuned out; otherwise, we would never be able to concentrate and would probably go insane. I believe, however, the mind never forgets anything but stores everything in what we call the subconscious. While undergoing hypnosis or brain surgery, we can recall or actually relive parts of our lives so precisely that we will remember things we never consciously remembered during the actual experience. The mind simply never forgets anything.

One of the first things I teach my classes is to get in touch with the wealth of information that the mind is processing. So many times I will ask a group how many deer they have seen, only to discover that not one person in the entire group has seen anything, though we may have passed within a few yards of scores of deer. I go on to explain that both they and I are bombarded by the same stimuli. The only difference is that I have taught myself to pay attention to the details that indicate deer are about. What they must do is get in touch with these details and nuances and thus enrich their observational skills. Their main problems are that their concentration is poor and that they have yet to learn what to look for.

All the information the student needs is stored in his subconscious, where it is sorted and retained. Only bits and pieces of vital information are passed on to his conscious mind. By relaxing and listening to his inner voice, he will open up the world of this stored information and even formulate some answers that will almost seem psychic. The subconscious can pick up fact A, then fact B, put them together like an algebraic equation, and send fact C to the logical conscious mind. Thus, the conscious mind may get the feeling it is being watched, but will not know why. The subsconcious has picked up slight movement A, as well as almost imperceptible sound B, then passed it on to the conscious mind in the form of feeling C: I am being watched. All the information is there; we just have to learn how to tap into it.

Grandfather would constantly urge us to go inside ourselves to check our perspective of the outside world. We would find that by relaxing, opening up to our inner voice, and listening, we would remember and feel things that we consciously missed. I remember lying back and relaxing after a long walk. Grandfather had asked us earlier if we had seen any deer, owls, foxes, or turkeys, and of course our answer was no. He then told us to go into ourselves and ask the deeper self what it had seen. Intuitively, I knew that I had passed a deer down by the place where the trail crossed the river and a fox den not far from that. I sensed these animals were there with no conscious evidence to substantiate what I had felt. Grandfather was delighted and took me back to the area, only to prove that the animals had been there, as the evidence of their tracks indicated.

He went on to explain that we had the same stimulation that he did, but our minds and thinking would not allow the information to get through. Slowly, over a period of many years, he nurtured our inner voices to the point where we would know and believe something just on gut feeling. We became so good at this that we took it for truth. Of course we proved the results time and time again, either through tracks, actual sightings, or other evidence, until it became a real part of our lives. In fact, our lives continuously revolved around not what we thought, but how we felt about something on a gut level. Beyond this obvious advantage, we began to feel the communication between ourselves and the natural world, with our inner instincts and intuitions acting as the interpreter. Our world blossomed, and we grew closer to the Earth because the Earth and we became of one mind.

To get in touch with the inner self, instincts, and intuitions, we first must define and feel the voice within. This voice comes to us in many ways, but it is universal to all people and can become a very powerful force in our lives if we will only take the time to learn how to use it.

The best way to describe this inner voice is through a passage from the book *Focusing* by Eugene T. Gendlin, Ph.D. "Our brains and bodies know far more than is normally available to us. We are conscious of only a fragment of what we deeply know. The central nervous system perceives and processes a great body of information that is stored outside the range of everyday awareness. Some of this information is best handled on an unconscious basis."

To get to this information, we must get in touch with our inner voice or "felt sense," which Gendlin describes as follows. "I can best describe it to you by starting with a familiar human experience: the odd feeling of knowing you have forgotten something but not knowing what it is. Undoubtedly, it has happened to you more than once. You are about to take a plane trip, let's say, to visit family or friends. You board the plane with a small, insistent thought nagging at you: You have forgotten something. The plane takes off. You stare out the window, going through various things in your mind, seeking that elusive little piece of knowledge. What did I forget? What was it?

"You are troubled by the felt sense of some unresolved situation, something left undone, something left behind. Notice that you don't have factual data. You have an internal aura, an internal taste. Your body knows but you don't.

"At some moments, the felt sense of what it is gets so vague that it almost disappears, but at other moments it comes in so strongly that you feel you almost know. Then suddenly, from this felt sense, it bursts to the surface. The snapshots! I forgot to pack the pictures I was going to show Charlie!

"You have hit it, and the act of hitting it gives you a sense of sudden physical relief. Somewhere in your body, something releases, some tight thing let's go. You feel it all through you: Whew!"

Simply stated, that tightness and loosening is the dynamics of your inner voice. That inner self never forgets anything and was screaming at you because it knew exactly what you had forgotten. The release came when your conscious mind finally remembered and the inner voice breathed a sigh of relief. The inner voice does not communicate in language but in mental pictures, images, dreams, visions, emotions, and inner feelings, to mention a few. At first, you will begin to work with the tightening and releasing concept until you become proficient and go on to more direct, less complicated forms of communication with the inner voice. The more you communicate the better you become and the more successes you will have. As I said, the inner self forgets nothing and is aware of the whole environment, as well as many of the things we can classify as nearly psychic. Tapping this wellspring means getting in touch with the inner voice, cultivating it, then using it every day. Once we learn how to ask it questions and interpret the answers, the results are nothing less than fantastic.

I had two medical students in my class who grew so proficient in the use of the inner voice that they took their final exam without studying. They used only their inner voice to answer the questions, believing that the inner self or subconscious never forgets anything. They aced the final. Another student who had lost a watch during a class the year before, found it by relying on her inner voice to guide her to the place where she had lost it. Other students can identify edible and inedible plants and their medicinal values by consulting their inner voice. I do caution strongly against this type of use unless you have a tremendous command of the plant world and many years of practice with the inner voice. Other students use the inner voice to find their way out of the woods, locate water, locate animals and good trapping areas, find edible plants, and discover answers to some serious questions in life. The successes are staggering, the failures few, the psychic ability phenomenal, and yet there is no scientific information as to why or how it works.

Asking and Utilizing the Inner Voice

The most important thing, after you know how to get in touch with the inner voice, is how to ask it questions in the proper way. If the questions are asked in the wrong way, then the answers will be vague at best, and sometimes nonexistent. So the way that questions are put to the inner voice is important for clear answers, with clearer and quicker answers coming with plenty of practice. Eventually, it is not enough just to be in touch with the inner self and to ask it good questions. You must get so good that it becomes second nature; then no questions need be asked.

At first, the questions to the inner self should be well thought out and very precise. Nothing should be vague or left to chance. To get some answers, it may take quite a few questions, narrowing the field until the proper answer is reached. We must learn to define and understand the voice within, the voice that is felt as a certain tightness in the pit of the stomach or as the release of that tightness. The end result will be an overall feeling of release, relief, and rightness as you instinctively know your answer is correct. The best way to explain the inner voice and how properly to ask it questions is to give some examples of experiences my students have had. Their views are much better than mine because they have only been using this method for a short period of time, while I have been using it for many years. In other words, they are closer to the problem of learning then I am, and their experiences are easier to understand.

Kevin and Larry have been to several of my classes over the past few years and, during an advanced class, finally learned to contact their inner voices. The advanced class is a full survival class held in the dead of winter. The students are permitted to bring in nothing but some scant clothing, they must rely on the edible plants and animals of the area for food, and they must make their own shelters and fire. Both Kevin and Larry have excellent skills and did very well with all the necessities of survival during the week, except for hunting. During all their outings and hunting trips, they saw hardly any animals. The ones they did see were too far away for a shot. By midweek they grew very frustrated with their naïve hunting and awareness abilities, and that is when I taught them about the use of the inner voice.

After a few days of practice, they decided to put the inner voice to work on the hunting problem. They felt that their subconscious minds were picking up many nuances and clues telling the where-abouts of game that the logical mind was missing. Relying on this premise, they walked out a short distance from camp, then stopped and relaxed. They then formulated a question, "Where are the animals?" They began slowly to turn in a circle, the tightness in their centers finally relaxing when they faced one direction, tightening up again whenever they faced another. They then began to walk the woods, stopping frequently to consult their inner voices to make sure they were still headed in the right direction. They were determined not to look at the ground for animal signs because they wanted to depend solely on the inner voice and not let the logical mind play tricks on them. Their path led them into an area where it was the most unlikely to find any animals.

Just about ready to give up, they consulted the inner voice one more time. This time it led them to an old, abandoned, debris hut, halting them just a few feet away. They were both upset that the inner voice didn't work for them after having such success with it over the past few days. Larry, in anger, threw his rabbit stick hard against the old debris hut. Out ran nine red squirrels from the leaf cover, a cottontail scampered from out behind the shelter, and a small raccoon crashed through the door and into the thicket. From the trees above, a small screech owl flew out. The men were so astonished that they forgot they were hunting, celebrating their achievement by screaming for joy, alarming the whole camp and chasing some local deer from the deep brush twenty feet from the old shelter.

Their inner voices had picked up sensations of the area for several days, collecting and storing it but never passing the information on to their thinking minds. Even though they wanted to see animals badly and needed the meat, the information would not pass through or formulate any clues. For the first part of the week, with all the trips and many miles and hours of travel, they only had seen a handful of animals. Yet following their inner voices for just fifteen minutes, they had seen more animals than they ever dreamed possible in the conditions of the thick winter pinelands. Their inner voices came through with the information needed from past subconscious stimulation and directed them right to the animals.

Going on to a more psychic and instinctual level of using the inner voice, I find the experience of Barbara, one of my students, very enlightening. I was talking to a group of students about the inner voice when Barbara asked me if it would work for things that we did not know, or had no way of knowing. I explained that I felt the inner voice was connected to our instincts, the spirit that moves through all things, and nature itself, giving us information about things we could not have possibly known. In disbelief, she consented to work an experiment with me that would prove the inner voice knew far more than we ever realized and would show its greater potentials.

I sat Barbara down, quieted the rest of the group, and told her to relax deeply. This form of meditationlike relaxation is part of what we teach in the advanced classes because it opens a student more to the flow of Creation. With her eyes closed and her body relaxed, I placed a piece of a plant into her open hand. I then told her to ask her inner voice whether it was edible or not. She said that it was edible. I then asked her if it was medicinal or not, explaining that a plant could be edible but not medicinal or vice versa. She consulted her inner voice and said that it was also medicinal. I then asked her to consult her inner voice and ask herself that if it is truly medicinal, where it would feel good in her body. She sat for a long moment and finally said that it would feel good in her stomach.

She got all three questions correct, right down to the medicinal properties and what part of the body the medication would affect. Everyone believed, at first, that she had known the plant by feel, but I explained that the plant part was only placed in her open hand then taken away. It was also a very rare South American species that I had taken from my medicine bundle and she in no way could have known what it was. The group and I then spent the afternoon doing the experiment over and over again with local but unknown plants, always coming up with the right answers and much more information than could be found in books. The students didn't realize it at first, but they were in definite and dynamic communication with plants. **Note**: *I am strongly against the use of the inner voice to give information on plants or any other intake, without having proper identification guides along to prove the results. The logical mind sometimes interferes with the inner voice, gut feelings, or instincts and can distort the answer, which can be a deadly mistake.*

Essentially, the inner voice can be used for many things, more than I have room to give in this book. With practice and experimentation, the sky is literally the limit. The most important thing is that you will learn to use the inner voice to communicate with the entities of the Earth and grow closer than you ever have before. You will reach an understanding far greater than mere skills and techniques. You will reach the ultimate oneness we all seek, and know forever that you are not alone in the natural world.

Physical Techniques and the Differences of Plants

It is not enough to say that each plant is different and has its own power. It is obvious that the differences between plant species are extreme in some cases and subtle in others. I refer to the differences between the same species of plant. I do not believe that two plants are physically identical in any way. Their leaves and flowers are as individual as fingerprints, and their personalities are as varied as the whole human race. Each plant contains not only its own shape, form, and makeup, but also has its own power and personality gleaned from the very land and conditions under which it grows.

It is important for the herbalist to know the plant people and how they vary with the land. He must realize that the medicinal qualities of a plant will vary from region to region, soil to soil, and even between plants growing side by side in the same microregion. The differences cannot be learned from a book or by word of mouth but only through dedicated study of the plant and how it affects us. Each person responds differently to the medications and food values of plants. A good herbalist will know what plant is meant for each individual. Once again, this comes with years of experience and experimentation. Certainly, the differences are at most times very subtle, rarely dramatic; but in the intricate world of the plant people and how they affect us, it is worth investigating.

Not only does each plant have individual qualities, but each phase of growth and part is different in the plant itself. For instance, the strawberry can be used as a food, tea, catalyst, or medication. Strawberries used only for medicinal applications can be harvested at various stages of its existence and external conditions; with each stage and condition, its medicinal value will change. Its dried leaves will be good for one thing, its green leaves are good for another. The medicinal values of the leaves are different than those of the flowers. There is also a variation of medicinal value within the stems, the young leaves, the seeds, and even within plants that grow in different soils. Young plants are different than young leaves, flowering plants are different than nonflowering, and leaves collected on a damp, misty morning are different than those collected on a warm sunny afternoon. Though slight, these differences are very important. Once again, experience and experimentation are the only teachers.

I have written this book to answer the questions of when to gather the plants and in what conditions they should be gathered.

The only time I make reference to the growth stage of the plant, the gathering conditions, or the soil in which they are found growing, is when that gathering technique will make a difference. Though much of what is contained in this book is general information, it lays the foundation for the exacting science of herbology and allows plenty of room for experimentation. With time, use, and the inner voice to direct the exact time and condition of collecting, the intimacies of each plant will be understood.

Collection, Preparation, and Storage

As I have stated, the stage of growth and condition of the plant when collected are very important to the medicinal and food values of the final product. When Grandfather sent us out to collect an herb, he would give us a very detailed description of what he needed, where it should be, its stage of growth, and the conditions under which it should be gathered. We would sometimes look for days, passing many of the plants in the process but never settling, always looking for the exact one he described. Many times we would have to let our hearts, or the inner voice, lead us to the proper location, especially when we were not blessed with an unlimited amount of time. It was not only important that the plant be gathered at the proper stage and conditions, but we had to gather the plant in the right way and in the sacred manner.

We always prayed before collecting and followed the sacred approach of making things right with our plant brothers, but the collecting went far beyond even that. When we collected the plants, great care was taken in its removal from life. It was always as if we were carrying the body of a beloved brother to his final resting place. We always expressed tremendous awe and respect for the plant's power. Some plants had to be gathered and gently wrapped in cloth, though others could be tied and hung upside-down; some roots could be left in the open, while others had to be kept in a cover of soil until needed. The way of gathering was as intricate and individual as the plant itself or its intended use. Eventually, all is learned through experience. However, the following are some general gathering techniques that can be used at first and are applicable to most plants.

Leaves, stems, and flowers can be gathered by taking the whole plant and cutting the stem from the root. These can be then tied at the stem bases in loose bundles and carried back to camp on the end of a long stick. For more careful collecting of leaves and flowers, select and pick them right off the plant and place them in a loose-weave bag, being careful not to pack tightly or crush in the transporting process. The whole flower can be picked or just the petals. Often I prefer the individual picking process because it doesn't kill whole plants and gives me the best leaves in the appropriate stage I need. Thus there is no waste and the plant still survives.

I gather roots by carefully digging them up, taking care not to bruise or cut into the root. I then place the roots in a basket and cover them with grasses or plant fiber to keep them out of the sun. Some roots are best kept covered in dirt until they are put in the root cellar or prepared for drying, but these will be mentioned individually later in the book. I try not ever to take a root without finding a use for the remainder of the plant. Nothing should ever be wasted; there is always a use if we look hard enough. I gather seeds, nuts, and the like by simply placing them into a basket or cloth bag, always leaving plenty to reseed or to feed my animal brothers and sisters.

There are a number of ways to prepare each plant for immediate or future use. Most plants that will be used immediately are used fresh and need little preparation. (Preparation of these plants either as a medicinal, catalyst, or food will be discussed in Part Two.) Some plants require intricate preparation processes, others need no preparation at all. Immediate or fresh-use plants are never stored for very long and are harvested as needed. Other plants can be prepared by drying. In some cases a tincture, pickling, or tea should be made, but these storage variations will be discussed in the main text for each individual plant.

Drying is quite easy, provided you don't do it too fast or under unfavorable conditions. Drying loosely wrapped bundles is easily accomplished by hanging them upside-down in a cool dry place. Depending on the conditions, the plants will be dry in about five to ten days. In most cases, the plants should crumble easily but never to a point of dust. Some plants should be a little pliable when the drying process is complete, but this is the exception and not the rule. (These exceptions will also be covered plant-by-plant.) Seeds, nuts, individual flowers, leaves, and stems can be spread on a wire or cloth mesh and laid out in mild sun every day, and then brought in at night to prevent the dew from spoiling the drying process. I find that hanging the mesh racks in a cool, dry place produces better results and does not reduce necessary medicinal qualities. Never dry over an open flame or woodstove, as this only drives away much of the medicinal value. Although thin roots can be hung to dry, thick roots should be sliced thin and dried on a rack, much like seeds.

The storage of plants is critical. To be lax on any phase of the preparation or storage of plants will severely diminish the medicinal value and lessen the shelf life. Many plants can be stored for long periods of time hanging upside-down in loose bundles. When some dried leaves or flowers are needed, simply break off from the bunch what you need and leave the rest hanging. Most seeds, nuts, flowers, leaves, and stems should be stored in loose-weave bags, hung from rafters in a cool and dry place. Bags should never be placed on shelves, as air cannot reach the bottom of the bag, and that may result in rotting. Earthenware or glass containers are also good storage receptacles. Plants should be broken up to the consistency of tobacco, and the lids should not be screwed tightly onto the jars, allowing some circulation. Never allow any stored plants to be in direct sunlight. Roots can be stored in loose bags, hung individually from rafters, or in containers. Steel or aluminum containers should never be used.

Herbology and the Herbalist

Many scientists, doctors, and lay people frown upon the ancient herbalist, believing his ways and medications are archaic, primitive, and noneffective at best. That line of reasoning is far from the truth, prepetuates a superstitious way of thinking, and gives all herbalists a bad name. Herbology is an exacting science as intricate as modern pharmacology. In fact, in ancient times, it took longer for a person to become an effective herbalist and healer than it does for a person to become a pharmacist or doctor today. Usually an individual was selected by the tribal medicine person when he or she was very young, then educated until middle age when he would take over from the healer as an herbalist. It wasn't until an herbalist was quite old and had numerous successes that he gained the respect of the tribe. You could become a doctor today in one-third the time.

Many of our modern medicines are still derived from herbs and nature. I'd have to write another whole book just to name all the ways plants are used today for medications, chemicals, and catalysts. Many of these medications were passed down from the ancients until modern times when scientists found a way to isolate and mass-produce a certain medication from the herbs. I still believe, when it comes to medication, that natural medications are better for the body than their synthetic counterparts, which give alarming side effects. I find, using my own body as a guinea pig, that the aspirin derived from the inner bark of red willow is far more effective than the store-bought type. It works faster, does not upset the stomach, and seems to control aches and fever far better.

The ancient herbalist did not just randomly mix up a concoction and give it to a patient. His time of gathering had to be precise. The preparation and storage of the plant had to be impeccable, and the mixing of the final herbal remedy had to be exact. An herbalist had his own mixing bowls and measuring devices so that he would know exactly the amount of the medicine reaching the patient without overmedicating him. He also had to know the patient well so as to prescribe the particular plant mixture that would integrate into the patient's life-style, body condition, size, and need. Unlike the modern medication meant for the masses, his science was exacting, intimate, and hard-learned through much trial and error, and ultimate successes.

Today, many herbalists do not take the time to learn their subject fully. They slip away into medication for the masses and wrongly try to replace modern doctors and medication, which we so badly need. Many modern herbalists have learned from books and, having little experience, they have the potential to hurt or kill someone. Many books out on the market today have herbal remedies that could actually poison or kill someone. One book described an Indian oral birth control preparation made from a particular plant. Anyone reading the book who knew anything about plants would have realized that the reason the birth control preparation worked was because the plant poisoned the woman's system so badly that she would not produce eggs, or at least not allow a fertilized egg to take hold. In many cases, with repeated use, the woman would become sterile or die.

There is no short-cut to becoming an effective herbalist. There are no books on the market that will replace a good teacher or medicine person, and there are no herbal teachers that can give to a student the vast amount of personal experience needed to become a good herbalist. Today, people want things fast and easy. They are not satisfied to work hard, observe carefully, and use themselves for experimentation by taking the time to feel what an herb does to their own bodies. Many people want to read and memorize the information it takes to become an herbalist, completely ignoring the intimacy and communication with the plant people, which is so necessary to becoming an effective herbalist.

Besides the wealth of knowledge passed on by his teacher and received through his experience, the ancient herbalist had to be a humanitarian, a psychologist, a friend, and a healer with a strong bedside manner. Knowing the patient was as important to the herbalist as was knowing the herbs and their worth. Not all herbal remedies would work on everyone equally, and thus an intimate knowledge of the patient's physical as well as spiritual makeup was necessary. Without this knowledge and the tremendous love that went with the craft, many of the herbal medications would not work.

I feel much the way the ancient ones did about the herbal remedies. If the Great Spirit put a disease on this Earth, he also put a plant or animal here to cure it. I believe that modern science has not yet fully tapped the vast knowledge of plants, and so much knowledge has been lost that it is almost irretrievable. So many old remedies and their catalysts, mixtures, and effects are buried in the past because no one listened or preserved this knowledge. Certainly, there are quacks in every profession, and the herbalists are no exceptions. The superstitions that some have created should be dispelled so that we can get on with new research.

The ancient herbalist was also his own laboratory. Herbalists knew their bodies so intimately that they would use them to test the effectiveness of herbal mixtures. Grandfather stressed this approach every time we sampled a wild edible food source. He would have us sit quietly, eat or drink the plant slowly, and feel with every fiber of our bodies the almost imperceptible changes and nuances the food would produce. We would totally sense the plant to a point where we were consumed by it, knowing it so intimately that it went beyond explanation. The body is one of the most important tools in the understanding and communication with the plant people. Savoring the food only brings it closer to the voice within.

Going Forward

I have written this book not only as a guide to edible and medicinal plants, but as an intimate account of the plant people as well. My hopes are to get away from the typical field guide and enter the secret world of plants, helping it to come to life in the reader's eyes. Becoming a good herbalist is hard work, and a good teacher or reliable book is needed before beginning. My hope is that this book will provide a starting point into the fascinating world of edible and medicinal plants. This book is only the first in a series that I hope will inspire the reader to go deeper into the study of plant people, rather than serve as just a superficial baptism. This book will become a doorway to greater things, and coupled with any of the great herbalists found around the world, modern man will be on his way to the ancient truths.

Caution

Because of the ever-increasing pollutants found in many soils, great care should be taken in gathering plants. Plants do not always filter out chemical pollutants, so it becomes necessary to take these precautions during the collecting process.

Never collect plants in or around any city, town, or highway, especially the areas along roadways and near factories; these areas are usually hazardous and full of pollutants. Never collect plants in any forestry area where cutting is going on or new forests are being planted. These areas are usually heavily sprayed with defoliants which could end up in the second generation plants. Be cautious around farm waste areas where chemicals could have been dumped, and stay away from any polluted or suspected polluted stream. Never collect near any kind of dump.

It is always best to collect in areas you know thoroughly. Wash all plants if you suspect any airborne pollutants could have drifted onto the leaves. Washing some leaves and other flower parts can remove the medicinal values. Always use the utmost caution in collecting any plants no matter what part you use. In the area you are collecting, check beyond the next rise or hedge to make sure there is not a surprise there, such as a polluting factory. Also keep in mind that some pollutants can change the medicinal values of plants.

Conservation

Although many plants grow in abundance across this country, there are some areas where a particular species does not flourish. In addition, there are plants that are on the endangered-species list throughout this country as a whole. In most cases I have only included those plants that grow in abundance throughout most areas of the country. I would suggest, however, that whenever you go out to collect a particular plant, you should check the plants in your state that might be on the endangered-species list. What may be abundant in one county may not be abundant in another. In many ways, it is up to us to make a conservation-based decision.

It was always Stalking Wolf's teaching, whether the plant was abundant or not, that we should always be instrumental in the propagation of these plants. We should especially try to propagate the least abundant plants whenever possible. We had to learn to look at all things as a gardener would look at his garden, for it was our sacred duty. In any area with any plant we gather, we should plant other seedlings or sow the seeds to insure that there will be more and healthier crops for the next season. It is especially important when dealing with endangered species. We should refrain from collecting them, but when we must, also insure that new seeds are properly planted.

We should learn all we can about the plants we will be collecting. This will aid us in the proper location of new plants and in our propagation processes. We must develop a deep love and respect for our plant brothers and take on the responsibility of the perpetuation of the species. We must also think of our grandchildren and the overall balance of nature to guarantee enough plants for upcoming generations. It is wrong to wipe all the plants of a particular species out of the area. Chances are they may come back only slowly or not at all. This is the blight that has hit our natural ginseng and so many other overused medicinal plants. We must use more forethought in our collection.

Grandfather had gardens all over the forests, fields, and swamplands, where he grew the herbs that he needed. That way he would not have to deplete the natural herbs and could grow his own healthy variety. Many times the seeds and cuttings from these gardens were transplanted to areas of the landscape that needed these plants badly. Many herbalists grow the natural edible and medicinal plants in their own home gardens for ease of collecting and to perpetuate an otherwise endangered species. Many people also plant abandoned fields with the natural vegetation. This is happening in the plains where concerned naturalists are trying to grow the original plants found on the ancient plains.

This "gardening" should not be done randomly or with little experience. It should be well thought out, especially where plants being cultivated will do the most good for not only the landscape but also for the animals. When I travel through the wilderness, a good portion of my job is to watch over nature's gardens, doing what I can to increase their numbers without killing off other plants. I hope the endangered-plant species will soon be a thing of the past so all people will be able to savor freely even the most uncommon plants. Until then, it will take a lot of work and dedication. What this society needs is more Johnny Appleseeds.

There is more to conservation than just the propagation of the plants we need for food, medication, or other utilitarian uses. It must become the propagation of all things, including animals. We must go about it not only with good intentions, but with a spiritual commitment and dynamic communication with the plants. We must understand that they are part of us and we of them. What we are looking for is a oneness with Creation so that we become an intricate part of the whole process. The more we get involved with the natural world, and the more we help out and become an intricate part of things, the more we understand, communicate, and feel our place in the world.

Science and the Mythical World of Plants

There is no denying the fact that for centuries, wild plants have helped heal the masses. In fact, just under 50 percent of our modern medication today comes from the plant people. One of the reasons plants helped heal people in the past was the placebo effect. This effect, which involved absolute trust in the doctor and his medication or just the plant itself, caused the body to heal itself. However, plants are far more than just placebos. Belief in the doctor and oneself are important, but the effects of plants can't be overlooked. Many of the ancient herbal remedies are full of powerful medications, and most have gone on to produce many modern drugs.

What is needed today is a more in-depth look at the healing herbs. It is not enough just to take a certain plant and analyze it, separating its certain components, and deeming them active or inactive. Many components of the plants work together; some are catalysts, some change when entering the body, some change with active ingredients, and of course, some are food. The time of year the herb is collected, the soil, and the weather conditions are all important considerations and should be included in any modern study. We cannot just pick up a plant and analyze it into neat little compartments. Modern science needs to listen to the old herbalists and their stories, study plants under all conditions, and come up with new, unprejudicial conclusions. What lies ahead is a vast area of science and the possibility of many new drugs and drug systems.

Certainly, there is not enough information or research done with the plant people and the old remedies to make any accurate judgment on their effectiveness. In many cases, plants have been found to have no discernible properties that give them medicinal values. Many of the modern scientists chalk the healing powers of plants up to superstition, and consider the ancient herbalists nothing but charlatans. Yet modern science continues to ignore the fact that up until 1975, about 75 percent of modern medications had absolutely no medicinal values, and are now considered placebos.

The placebo effect occurs when a patient believes so strongly in the drug or doctor that he activates and accelerates the healing process within the body. Generally 70 percent of the time we see a doctor for illnesses that need not be treated by modern medicine. This, of course, is not to say that doctors are unnecessary and we should cut down on the visits to the modern office, but in many cases our illnesses are self-curable. I believe that any over-the-counter medication that we get from the pharmacy can be replaced by its suitable plant counterpart. For more serious illnesses, I strongly suggest going to the doctor, as the intricate preparation of the more advanced plant medicinals take time and exact measurements. They could, in the hands of the untrained, become potentially dangerous, especially in the area of overmedication.

The Power of Plants

I strongly believe that if the Creator put a disease on this Earth, there is a plant that was put here to cure it. We have lost much of our inherited plant knowledge due to poor records, lack of interest, and the advance of modern medications. We can never truly recover that knowledge, and we are in danger of losing even more if we don't take an active interest in the preservation. I believe that modern science hasn't even scraped the surface of the plant medicinal potential but I see a trend toward more research in the area. We should help the preservation process by actively seeking out our elders and learning what they have to teach.

This book is written primarily for those of us who can't get to a doctor or a pharmacy. To pure survivalists or people actively involved in long trips out into the wilderness, we must do as our ancestors did. We must learn to take care of ourselves by utilizing the viable medicinal and edible plant resources so abundantly available to us. It is also written for those people who are tired of manufactured nonprescription synthetic drugs and their unnatural side effects. We are looking for more natural alternatives that have little or no side effects and are more in line with a holistic life-style. In the long run, the natural medications are far better for the body than the synthesized garbage we buy over the counter, and in my studies, more effective.

The power of the natural plants cannot be overlooked or passed off as some placebo. I find that the aspirinlike substance found in certain willow barks works better and faster than the manufactured aspirin or its substitutes. It also has far less side effects and does not upset the stomach. Scientific investigation into that particular species of willow confirms that the inner bark does contain aspirinlike substances and that it is as effective as aspirin. The problem lies, however, in the way we obtain, prepare, and measure the substance.

Certainly, going to the store and buying nice, little aspirin tablets and capsules is easier, but not better. I believe that the whole process of obtaining natural medications is better for you in the long run. You have to be out in the pure and natural world, looking for the plant. This in itself cuts down on stress and its related illnesses so, in point of fact, you need far less aspirin. The meticulous care and preparation of the plant also adds to a sense of relaxation and the confidence in knowing that you can do things for yourself. Finally, when it comes time to prepare the medication, you give yourself or your patient the exact amount needed to do the job.

Problems with plant medications usually stem from improper collecting, preparation, or dosage. You can just as easily overdose yourself with plant medications as you can with the regular non-prescription drugs. The improper time of collecting or poor preparation and storage can also render a plant useless, inactive, or weak in medicinal values. It is extremely important to know what you are doing in all phases of preparation and dosage. In the past, pseudo-herbalists have passed down misinformation and caused much pain and suffering. This has encouraged skepticism within the world of modern science.

Wild plants as a food source become even more important and better for one's overall health. We eat too many processed foods and are saturating our bodies with far too many chemicals which we hardly know anything about. Natural- and health-food centers are one alternative, but they are usually expensive because of the short shelf life of the products and the costs of organic gardening. What we have for the taking outside our doorsteps is the biggest and most inexpensive of all health-food markets. Instead of the long drive to the market, we can gather in warm sunlight and refreshing breezes, while taking long walks and blending in beautifully with the natural world. Thus, the overall benefit of the food is increased by the healthy way we have to collect the plants.

The food value of wild plants, in my experience, is far better than anything you can find in a supermarket. The other minerals, vitamins, and compounds found in them tend to round out our diets. Wild plants are always fresh and definitely the healthiest of all foods. If collected correctly, they contain little pollutants and have none of the preservative chemicals used in commercially prepared food to extend shelf life. I think that a big part of Grandfather's long life can be attributed to his way of using the natural world and the various cycles of food.

During the spring, summer, and fall, I rarely saw Grandfather sit down to a meal. Instead he would be constantly foraging for food, nibbling on fresh and healthy tidbits as he went on his way. To him the natural world was like living in one huge supermarket: Everything was there for his taking. His way of life was the healthiest I have ever seen, and I cannot remember ever seeing him sick. When I met Grandfather I was seven years old, and he was eighty-three. He never faltered in hiking, climbing, or swimming, nor showed any signs of old age. He was always active, and his mind was always clear and sharp. Today, at thirty-five years old, I am not nearly as active as he was at eighty-five. As I grew within modern society, my body has degenerated and my energy has waned. But I have learned a valuable lesson and am actively on my way back to using natural plants as my prime food source.

I remember once passing a nursing home with Grandfather. We looked upon the old and forgotten, those who had lost their self-esteem and purpose in life and were feeble of mind and body. Ironically, most of those people were at least ten years Grandfather's junior, yet they seemed so dead. Grandfather only shook his head in disgust and commented that these old ones were there because of inactivity and a lifetime of poor diet. "What good is living to old age," he said, "if you can't enjoy all the potential activities that go with that freedom." Modern science proclaims longer overall lives, but at what cost and quality? I'd rather be dead at sixty-five than be among the living dead at eighty.

I am not denouncing modern drugs, doctors, or foods any more than I am denouncing the old ways. I believe that we can strike a balance between old and new, reaching new levels of health in body, mind, and spirit, and living to an active old age. Each side has to lose the cynicism toward the other, acquiring a balanced harmony of existence. We can't fight with the old and the new but must learn from them both, incorporating them into a more viable life-style that is close to the Earth. Prejudice and tunnel vision are our biggest obstacles in this marriage. Both new and old studies are for the betterment of mankind, but they fall short of that goal in their fight to prove the other wrong.

I find this same fight in so many other areas of life. It becomes especially apparent between those people who are fighting to save the Earth and the old ways. It seems that no two groups can agree with each other or the methods that this overall saving task must take. Instead they fight with each other and burn up energy while remaining at a standstill with their common goal. What we need are people with visions that overlook the petty differences, keeping their energies focused on the larger battles. We must have all people come together no matter the color, race, or religion if we are to save what we have left. We are all people of the Earth and there is no real turning back, so why not work side by side in the awesome battle to save the Earth. For if one fails, we all fail.

We also have a greater responsibility when using wild plants for medication or food. We have the responsibility to conserve and propagate whenever possible, keeping in mind the other animals and generations of people that will utilize the plants. We must be careful to make the right choices and ensure a healthy future in all worlds. We are the caretakers and must never take more than the land can bear, or become so full of greed that we forget those who follow.

Healing

The process of being a healer in the physical sense is as demanding as knowing the plants. I believe that for one to become a good herbal healer there must be a firm foundation of basic truths common to all who seek this path. First of all, the healer must be one with the Earth. He has had to find the time to understand himself through the eyes of nature, learning who he is and where he fits in. He has had to break down the barriers that keep him separated from the natural world so that there is no inner or outer dimension. His prime source of understanding and knowledge must come to him from the Earth, and he must realize that he is nothing more than a hollow vessel that the Earth uses to heal.

The healer understands that Earth is his true mother and all things that keep him alive come from Mother. He treats all entities of the Earth as true brothers and sisters, for they also call Earth their mother. Kinship with all things is a real part of his existence, and he has come to know the entities of the Earth as his personal friends, teachers, and constant companions. He is never alone, for all of Creation speaks, and he is always in communication with the Creator. The people of the Earth are also his brothers and sisters, fathers and mothers, grandfathers and grandmothers, for they all come from one family. The terms grandfather and grandmother not only denote that kinship, but also display the fact that a teacher is called by this title because he has the years and experience, no matter what the age.

The healer does not seek out external possessions as his foundation. His is a world of peace, love, and joy found within himself. He understands that all people, no matter what they do, are trying to seek out that peace, love, and joy, but are distracted by trying to find it externally. Though the healer may be very wealthy or a poor ascetic, he does not cling to the artificial or gear his life to the world of possessions. Anyone, no matter what the life-style, can be a powerful healer if his heart is full of peace, love, and joy, and he is one with the Earth—brother or sister to all.

A healer is a believer in life. He believes that disease is just a disharmony in life. He seeks the truth but realizes that many truths cannot be proven. Faith is his biggest ally. To him the Earth is a bountiful mother, and all the things needed to preserve a healthy life for him or his patient are always there. He listens with his heart not with his head, and he truly cares for people. He loves his enemies, for he believes that no matter what you send out, so too will you get in return. Hatred and greed are foreign to him and he seeks to fight that negativity with love and understanding. Though he is peaceful, he is also a warrior, defending what is right with force if necessary. He is not led to battles as a lamb to slaughter. He can also see both sides of any story, becoming at most times a mediator.

His care toward the land and his brothers and sisters is a powerful driving force. He is not only a healer of people but a healer of animals, plants, and Earth. This caring can be seen in his tremendously soothing bedside manner. His power can be felt in the love he has for his patient and the faith he has in the Creator. There is no such thing as bad luck, only good teachers. He not only tries to correct the symptom and illness, but also to reach the bad medicine that originally started that illness. His is the way of the Earth, and the Earth is his source of power. Helping people does not tire him but exhilarates him. His many fights to preserve that which is pure and natural are draining. Any healer that looks well rested is not doing his job.

The healer knows his patient well, getting to know him far better than a brother. He listens and says little for he must base the preparation and dosage of the herbs he is using on that particular patient. He derives those dosages as much from the heart as he does from knowledge. He realizes that he is nothing more than an understanding placebo, and the power to heal comes from the plant, the Creator, and the patient himself. He knows when to back away and allow modern medicine to take over. He is not prejudiced and skeptical but marvels at the modern wonders and tries to integrate both whenever possible. Even with patients under care of a doctor and commercial drugs, he is still there with his powerful bedside manner. His ego is not damaged, for all he is interested in is the patient's health.

The medicinal properties of the wild edible plants found in this book and the dosages are for the average person. There is great variety in the choices and even ways of increasing the dosages. Remember, however, that certain conditions should not be treated with natural medications and medical advice should always be sought out. This is not to say that the plants are ineffective, but rather the preparation and dosage may demand more than your skill can afford. Go to your doctor for more serious maladies unless you are in a survival situation where prompt medical attention or modern drugs are not available. This book is written from my experience, and I am not prescribing any plant as a medicinal or edible. What may be good for the masses may affect an individual adversely because of allergies. Start with little doses and watch the body's reaction.

How to Use This Book

This book is not a field guide to the identification of wild edible or medicinal plants. Nor is it a book of prescriptions using wild plants. I do not recommend this book as a pharmacy alternative or as a substitute for modern medical therapy. Instead, it is a book about plants and the intimate knowledge that I have gathered over years of experience. The medications are ones that I have learned and used in survival situations when getting to a doctor or pharmacy was impossible. Even though the plants prescribed have gone through extensive field testing by myself and countless students, I do not recommend them as medicinals. It takes far too much practice and time to understand the principles of modern herbology and its many variations.

Use this book as a back-up to your field identification guides. My ambition is to bring the reader or student survivalist closer to an intimate understanding of our plant brothers. I also hope to clarify some of the misconceptions about the plants and their uses by showing the close relationship the native people have with all the entities of the Earth. Through this book, I also hope to teach a deeper understanding and reverence for the Earth and a deeper communication with our Mother. In essence, this book is a book of introduction, an introduction beyond the superficial world of names and scientific classification. It is a world of real spirits and entities as rich in lore as any other facet of nature.

PART TWO

Amaranth (*Amaranthus hypochondriacus*)

Description   Amaranth is a stout, weedlike, annual herb, six inches to six feet tall. Stems are rough, hairy, and freely branching. Leaves are usually three to six inches long, alternate, toothless, rough and veiny, ovate to lanceolate. The undersides of young and lower leaves are purple. The amaranth flowers grow in green axillary clusters up to two-and-a-half inches long. Seeds abound, shiny black, in chaffy bracts at the ends of stems and branches. Its roots are red. Amaranth may be found in waste ground and disturbed soils. With the exception of desert and alpine areas, amaranth grows through the northeast section of the United States, south to Florida, and west to the Pacific states.

Personality   Whenever I encounter amaranth during my outings, I am taken back to the time I met this soothing but powerful spirit. Stalking Wolf, Rick, and I were on our way to our base camp, when we passed a rather large patch of our amaranth brothers. Stalking Wolf motioned to us to stop and sit. He began to speak to the eldest plant, asking permission to use some of the plant people for food and medicine. As soon as Rick and I heard his words, we instinctively knew that we were about to learn something important. We sat nearby, reverent for the prayer and the death which was about to take place, while remaining attentive to everything he might say about this plant. As he spoke to the plant, he caressed the leaves with his hands, sniffed the seed heads, and lovingly admired its beauty. He stood pausing for a long moment, eyes closed, as if he were feeling the spirit of the plant flow through him and become part of him.

After placing an offering of sacred tobacco at the foot of the eldest plant, he carefully began his work, without touching that plant again. Gently, he began to gather the seeds, shaking the seed heads inside his buckskin bag until most of the seeds were removed. He was always careful not to take them all because many birds and animals use this plant for winter food. He always taught us to consider our other brothers and sisters whenever we take anything from the landscape. Saying a prayer for health and for fast growth, he then carefully planted some of the seeds around the larger plant bases to insure that there would be a healthy population of amaranth next season. He did not gather from any of the large and strong plants, for he knew they were needed to produce seed for the winter.

He then, with reverence, began to select a few of the most succulent leaves from each plant, putting them into the buckskin bag along with the seed. For him, the act of breaking leaves off a plant was not unlike ripping the limbs from an animal; all spirits are equal. Stalking Wolf was careful to remove only a few leaves from each plant so this would not hinder its growth and longevity. Without explaining what the plant was to be used for, he asked us to study the plant, its growth, and position in the landscape. He did this often as a way of making us aware how each plant or animal fit into the ecosystem. We knew from past experience that we should look for animal signs and tracks around the base of these tall and beautiful plant people. This would tell us what animals depended on the plant for cover, shade, or food. A deeper look enabled us to discover what other plants grew beside and intermingled with the amaranth. We then tried to understand their relationships. Again, we were reminded that it wasn't important just to know the plant was edible and medicinal, but to understand how the plant fit into the landscape and related to the animal people.

Back at camp, Stalking Wolf began to teach us about the leaves of the amaranth. Each holding a leaf in our hands, we instinctively knew that it was edible; but Stalking Wolf asked us to go deeper and reach out with our feelings to see if we could feel the medicinal power of the plant. Though he did not deny us the use of our plant identification books, he tried to lead us to a greater understanding of a plant through intuition and instinct. For him, there must be a real bond between man and plant, a brotherhood, a communication beyond words. Man must know a plant on all levels just as he would know his best friend. This brought us closer to the essence of the spirit that moves through all things: no inner or outer dimension, no separation of man and plant, but a oneness.

Stalking Wolf proceeded to boil the leaves of the plant with the care of a master chef. He sniffed the steam and instructed us to do the same. Each plant was to be savored and remembered, just as the finest wine is appreciated by a wine taster. Holding a cup to us in the firelight, Stalking Wolf asked us to sample this mild medication for soothing the stomach. With the utmost respect, appreciation, and reverence, I felt the hot, mildly astringent liquid trickle down my throat and leave a soothing, warm coating deep within my stomach. The same slow, methodic procedure was used in eating the leaves, which were delicious, powerful, and very filling. It was a strict rule that we ate slowly, so that we did not eat more than was necessary, and enabled ourselves to savor and enjoy the plant and begin to know its spirit. Stalking Wolf felt that modern man ate his food too quickly, which produced obesity and a loss of sensitivity to taste, causing most people to miss the real pleasure of food.

Later that evening, we laid the seeds on top of a flattened log, placing it near the fire. We parched the seeds slowly, stirring them often so that they were evenly cooked. The next morning, Stalking Wolf spread out a blanket and placed the parched seeds into the center. Holding a palmful of seeds high in the air, he began to rub them gently in his palms. The wind carried the chaff off, dropping the seeds onto the blanket. In a short time, we had a huge pile of black, shiny seeds. We put these seeds into a log pot, added water, and proceeded to rock boil them. Near the end of the boiling process, as the seeds thickened into a cereal, Stalking Wolf added some roots of sassafras to add a distinct flavor. The cereal was wonderfully filling. We did not have to eat again until dark.

I have learned much about my amaranth brothers over the years, both from watching Stalking Wolf and using my own instincts about the plant. I have grown to know it as a brother. I believe the more I use a plant, the more instinctively I know about it. Its essence and spirit become part of me. My first and most valuable lesson about the plant's healing spirit was during a late summer survival outing with Rick and Stalking Wolf. Rick had diarrhea and bad abdominal cramps, which had the potential of calling off our survival experience prematurely. Stalking Wolf disappeared for a short time returning with some old, but green amaranth leaves. Placing the leaves in a pot, we boiled them rapidly for quite a while until most of the water had evaporated. He then gave Rick a cupful to drink. The cramps disappeared almost immediately, and within a few hours the diarrhea subsided. Rick felt the medicinal power of the plant while it saturated his entire body, working in a warm, soothing way on his digestive system. The warmth stayed with him for hours.

Food   The amaranth is one of my favorite wild edible plants. One of the most delicious parts of the amaranth is its soft, fleshy top. I boil these until they are almost tender, much like broccoli would be prepared. Some people prefer to boil them to a softer consistency, but that depends on how you prefer your vegetables. In a survival situation, I most often use a steam pit for amaranth tops. This helps to hold in much more of the flavor. At home I like to eat them with butter or cover them with melted cheese as a vegetable substitute for the evening meal.

The young and succulent leaves are best eaten raw or added to a salad. At home, they are especially delicious when mixed with scrambled eggs and cooked. Add mushrooms to this concoction to put a taste of the wild into your morning. The older, green leaves can be cooked like spinach by steaming or boiling. I find that the older amaranth leaves make a great spinach substitute for any spinach recipe. I make a habit of saving the water that is used to boil the amaranth, as this can be used later for medication taken internally or used externally.

In a survival situation, I simply winnow the seeds by rubbing them between my palms over a blanket. The chaffs are carried away by the winds. For home use, I use winnowing baskets and trays. The seeds can then be parched and ground into flour or simmered into a cereal. On occasion, I add wintergreen berries, sassafras roots, or honey directly to the cooking cereal to add a light, aromatic sweetness. I also sprinkle unground amaranth seeds atop my breads and cereal to add a crunchy, nutty flavor. One of my favorite breads is made by using a recipe of one-third amaranth flour, one-third acorn flour, and one-third whole wheat flour, adding water, and making ash cakes. Ash cakes are simply flattened, pancaked dough laid on the white, hot wood ash of campfires, turned frequently to cook evenly. Surprisingly, the ash cakes pick up relatively little ash residue, and are delicious with honey, home preserves, wild berries, or maple syrup. Amaranth seeds make good stew and soup thickener. Many farm researchers are now looking into amaranth as an alternate cultivated grain because the seed heads can contain thousands of seeds and the plants need very little cultivation.

Warning: *I must caution the use of amaranth in suspected pollution areas, as the plant easily picks up and accumulates high levels of nitrates. This can cause severe gastrointestinal discomfort, cramps, and nausea. This caution stands for both the edible and medicinal uses.*

Medicinal   The medicinal properties of the amaranth are as varied and powerful as the edible ones. A mild to strong tea can be used as an effective treatment for diarrhea and other gastrointestinal disorders. The strength of the tea is determined by the severity of the diarrhea. I have also seen people use the tea to slow an excessive menstrual flow. A mild to medium-strong tea can be used as a gargle for mouth and throat irritations. I have found it very effective for soothing cold sores and sore throats due to colds and flus. A mild to strong tea makes an effective astringent for all types of skin wounds, sores, pimples, insect stings, and poison ivy irritation. Generally, it is a great medication for internal and external wounds.

The proper medicinal preparation of the freshly gathered amaranth is not as difficult and time consuming as most others. The boilings saved from the making of foods are sufficient and suitable for medication as previously described. Generally, the strength or weakness of the tea is judged by color, and boiling tends to dissipate much of the medicinal powers. I usually start out with a weak tea for most maladies and ask the people who seek my advice on medicinal plant uses to do the same. If the strength is not sufficient in alleviating the illness, then increase the dosage or strength of the tea. Usually, one cup of medium strength tea is sufficient for most internal illnesses.

When I gather and store the amaranth plant for winter use, I am careful of its preparation and drying. I gather the newest, most tender, succulent green leaves from near the center of the amaranth, usually two days after a rain. I hang them in loose bunches in a cool, dry place and allow them to dry thoroughly. I then break up the leaves into a tobaccolike consistency and store them in earthenware or wooden containers (glass is a fine substitute). In mixing the tea for medicinal use, I add a palmful (about one ounce) to an eight-ounce cup of water. Some of the medicinal property is lost upon drying, so I increase my dosage to two cups a day for any internal malady. I have not known anyone to be allergic to amaranth, but will suggest to a first-time user of this as a food or medication that you use only a little at a time until you know your system can tolerate it.

We must use care not to deplete an entire area of amaranth or any other plant. The seeds that may stay on the amaranth plant until early spring will be used by the birds and animals for their own winter survival.

Angelica (*Angelica archangelica*)

Description Angelica is a member of the parsley family. The flowerheads of angelica are like exotic greenish-white clouds suspended on an arrangement of stems resembling a Tiffany setting. The stem is dark purple and very smooth, reaching a height between four and nine feet. Most of the upper leaf stalks have a bladderlike basal sheath, while the lower leaf stalks usually have peeled back theirs. The stalks support three leaflets which can be further divided into three to five more leaflets. The angelica favors streambanks, swamps, and wetlands, growing sometimes in huge rafts, adding their whiteness to the otherwise monotonous green swamplands. The name *angelica*, which means "angellike," conjures up exotic, heavenly thoughts of its rich past. It flowers from late June to mid-October, depending on the area. It is a plant of the Northeast, ranging from eastern Canada, south to Delaware, and as far west as Illinois.

Personality Stalking Wolf cautioned us as he introduced us to the angelica growing along the water. He said that this plant is a very powerful healer from the water's edge, but must never be confused with the poison water hemlock and its relatives. For us, the plant held a certain mystique, especially in the set of its flowerhead, as if a cloud of green were suspended on a minute, multifaceted setting. I don't know whether it was the exotic look of the plant, its close resemblance to the poisonous water hemlock, or the power of its spirit, but it captivated us beyond words.

We lay on the spongy banks of the river for a long time, looking up at the sea of green lacy flowerheads, feeling a certain refreshing coolness amid the raft of angelica. I felt as if I were in a room separated from the rest of the river and forest, a room of soothing green, a cathedral within a cathedral. The elegant tapestry of leaves and the deep purple stems added a surrealistic imagery to the whole experience, transcending common consciousness. I was totally enraptured in angelica elegance even before I realized its power.

Stalking Wolf took us beyond the boiled, earthy tastes of the edible roots that we knew so well as a survival food. Using the medicinal power of the plant that day, we unlocked the soothing essence we found lying under those plants. We found that the plant contained within its core the same soothing power that we could tap at will—a power that could reach deep into our bodies.

The preparation of the angelica root was almost a religious experience to Stalking Wolf. The whole process seemed to be slow

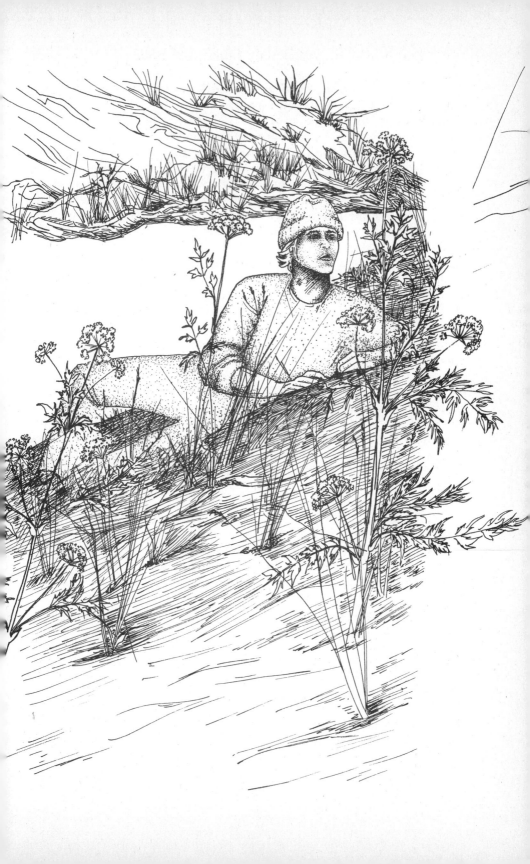

and relaxed, very introspective. Carefully, a freshly dug root was laid bare of its rough coat, its core cupped in his rough hands and held up to his nose to smell its essence. Long pauses between procedures were the rule; prayer and words of love muttered under his breath produced a certain melodious drone. The root was gently cut apart and placed into a pot of rapidly boiling water where it then steeped for over an hour. The pot was watched and smelled frequently to catch the brew at just the right time. Stalking Wolf said that I could not see or smell when the tea was just right, I had to feel it, assimilate its relaxing power from within.

I raised the cup of tea to the light and gazed deep into its inner power. The tea was deep and strong, yet gentle to the eyes and nose. I drank slowly and thoughtfully, following the slow ritual as taught by Grandfather. I felt the tea slowly warm my throat, stomach, then lower bowels. A deep soothing feeling came over my center and reached outwardly, relaxing even the extremities of my body. The cramps I had experienced earlier and throughout that day disappeared, and I slept a profound, angelica sleep.

Food   The angelica root should be harvested in late spring or early fall, when it has the most nutritional value. The roots should be carefully peeled and boiled until tender. It can then be eaten like a boiled potato or added to stews. I have found it helpful to know the withered winter skeleton of the angelica, which guides me to the root during the lean months. Usually, because the angelica is located near streams or swamps, the ground is not frozen during the winter months, thus allowing an easy harvest.

My first taste of angelica roots came during a weekend survival campout in the northern Pine Barrens. Magically, Stalking Wolf began gathering angelica roots in an old swamp. There was hardly anything left of the angelica skeleton, but he knew the plant so well that even the stubble indicated to him where the roots were located. I caution anyone but an expert to use just the stubble or withered winter skeleton as a primary indicator of angelica root, because it is very closely related to the poison water hemlock.

After the roots were gathered and peeled, we boiled them for a little over an hour by our meager campfire, on an icy bank overlooking the swamp. The cold was numbing and the dampness bit to the marrow of our bones. We shivered because our bodies were long without food. Those first few angelica roots were absolutely delicious. Warm and tender, they quickly filled the hollowness of our hunger and gave us strength to go well into the night before making camp.

It wasn't until the next season that we knew the plant upon whose roots we had feasted.

Caution: *Again, I must emphasize the necessity of using a reliable field guide in identifying the angelica, as it is very closely related to the poisonous water hemlock.*

Medicinal The medicinal uses of angelica are as soothing and exotic as its nature. The absolute calming reverence Stalking Wolf felt for the plant was enough to teach me its overall effectiveness as a powerful medicine. Eating the plant's roots alone is not enough of a baptism to feel its essence; instead, one must view the plant from another perspective. Illness or internal discomfort provides that other perspective, for it teaches one the soothing power this herb has within its roots and seeds.

Generally, I make a number of teas from the various parts of the plant. The strongest and most powerful tea comes from the crushed seeds. A small palmful of powdered seeds (about one tablespoon) is added to a cup of boiling water and allowed to stand for thirty minutes. The liquid is then warmed again and drunk as a tea. Weaker teas are made from the root that has been gathered in the spring, peeled, dried, and powdered. Powdering is not necessary, but more steeping time is needed when using fresh root or chunked dried root. A small palmful of the powdered root is added to a cup of boiling water and allowed to steep for five to fifteen minutes, depending on the strength needed. Fresh root tea can be extracted during the root cooking process and used at a later date or immediately for an ailment. The intensity of the ailment will indicate what strength tea to use.

Teas made from the seeds are very powerful and can be used for severe cramps, vomiting, or stomach upset. I have also used them during survival trips to soothe the ulcers of a few of my students who had forgotten their ulcer medications; they had better results than with their regular medication. Teas made from the roots will relieve mild cramps and other digestive disorders as well as stimulate appetite and induce kidney function. A half cup twice a day is a good dosage for any of the above maladies.

Root teas of the stronger varieties have a calming effect and have produced good results in relieving tension headaches. I also used a combination of the root and seed teas to help fight a fever during a recent illness. The tea had a tremendous calming effect and lowered my fever and relieved my headache. Because I have found that angelica tea is great for the common cold, I use it quite a bit during the regular school winter survival trips when colds are common. I have had great results using crushed angelica roots for the relief of itching and as a general hand lotion, especially in winter when hands are subject to cracking and chafing.

Large doses of the teas can have an effect on the heart rate, blood pressure, and respiration. I suggest that one use caution in the use of these teas, as overmedication can be dangerous. Leave the stronger doses of teas to the well-trained herbalist and not to the beginner.

Roots should be collected in middle to late spring. They should be peeled, thinly sliced, and dried in the sun, much like dried fruit is prepared. Make sure that the slices are fully dry and of a brittle texture. This will make grinding and powdering easier. The roots should then be ground using the ancient stone-grinding method, mortar and pestle, or a modern grinder. Powder should be spread out and allowed to dry again to insure that no moisture remains. I do not recommend drying the slices in a commercial food dryer because this quick-drying process destroys much of the medicinal value of the plant.

Seeds are collected when they turn brown. I spread them in a large tray or put them on a screen in the sun. Make sure that the seeds are totally dry. Do not use a fire or parch the seeds as the excess heat diminishes the medicinal values. Once the seeds are dry, grind them as you would do for the roots, then let them dry once again in the sun. Store both the dried powdered seeds and roots in glass or earthenware containers in a cool dry place. If stock smells moldy or rancid, discard, as the powder has gone bad due to moisture.

Black and White Birch (*Betula lenta and B. papyrifera*)

Description   Birch trees are quite tall, ranging between forty-five and seventy feet. They are usually very straight trees with white to dark brown or black bark. The newer bark hugs the tree tightly and is marked by the horizontal scarlike stripes common to most birches. The broken twigs of the birch, especially in early spring, have a wintergreenlike odor. The leaves can be one to five inches in length and are beautifully elliptical with serrated edges. Flowers are produced in late spring. The fruits, in mid-fall, are eaten by many song and game birds. Several mammals consume the succulent bark and twigs. Black birches are found in mature forests from Ontario to as far south as Delaware and west to Ohio. They reach down into Georgia via mountain ranges. The white birch also is found in the northeast corner of the United States and east to Illinois.

Personality   The Pine Barrens are dotted throughout with the white birch, but one small grove in particular has always intrigued me. As far back as I can remember, I visited this little grove, climbing in the branches, jumping from tree to tree, or nestling down on the yellow bed of fall leaves strewn on autumn's forest floor. Going into the little birch grove was like visiting some strange ivory temple, the pillars of white and translucent green leaves reaching up to blue skies. The leaves shimmered in light wind like no other tree my young mind had ever known. The place was wild and magical, always drawing me close throughout the year.

Stalking Wolf introduced me to this place. I remember the reverent intonations and words he used in the description and introduction of these tree people to me. There the feelings of awe and magic started, but the underlying quality of the area reached out to me on deeper levels. I used to marvel at the elegance and grace of these trees. Some, bent by winter's heavy snows, bowed their heads to the Earth as if in respect of some unseen spirit. Even in their bowed position, there was still that certain gracefulness that could not be overlooked.

This grove of trees was always dancing, not only with shimmering leaves but with whirling tree tops. The bent trees appeared as if they were going through some eloquent choreography known only to the Creator. I always made it a point to visit this little grove whenever there was a storm raging. Either sitting in the uppermost branches violently swaying with the trees or watching from afar, I

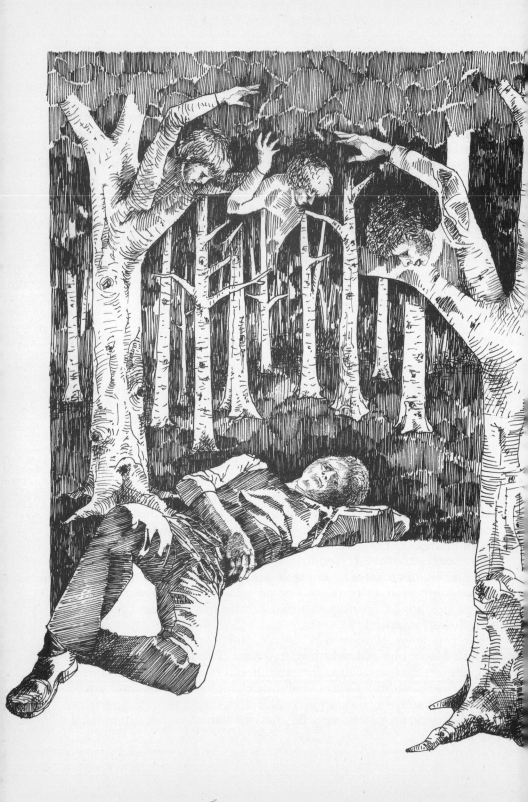

could not help getting caught up in the grand dance of wind, leaf, and tree. The totality of movement and flow was easily internalized, and suddenly the spectator became a participant.

I guess it was Stalking Wolf's intention to let me play with the trees and know them as friends and brothers before he began to teach me of their foods and medications. So many times he would acquaint me with things to know about them for no other purpose than to enjoy their uniqueness and splendor, finally adding the dimension of utilitarianism only after he was satisfied that I loved for the sheer pleasure of being close. The introduction to the functional uses of the birches was slow and methodical. It began first with a small twig of birch placed in my mouth, where I savored its taste and aromatic qualities. With that first lesson and the strange, good taste in my mouth running through my body and linking me to the tree's essence, I could not help but feel part of the trees.

I remember the first cup of birch tea very well. A cold winter wind had snapped off one of the upper branches of the larger birches. During a winter walk, we found it lying on the ground. Grandfather thanked the forest for the much-needed gift and turned away to the grove's edge to build a fire. When the water boiled, he added a handful of tiny twigs and bark shavings and let it steep for near a half hour. That tea was delicious, warming, and so damn appreciated during that frozen part of the year. I felt warmer than I would have with regular tea. There was a tremendous sense of summer to the taste.

I can't drink a cup of birch tea today without thinking back to the fantasy of the little grove. That grove has fallen to the bulldozer, but the memories still hang strong in my mind. Campouts there were so magical, carefree, and full of excitement. All sorts of animals used the area for fun it seemed, the little birch grove drawing from all over the landscape. So many lessons were learned there on the edge of the forest. So much beauty, elegance, and goodness come from our birch brothers.

Food I've savored the rich taste of birch syrup on ash cakes or acorn bread so many times. One of our many rituals in the spring was to tap the rich supply of sap from the birch groves. One huge tree in particular produced the best of all syrups, sweeter than any other tree I have yet tapped to this day. It was an old friend, probably reaching back a few hundred years, located on what was once an old homestead. The tap marks still remain and can be reused year after year without disturbing the tree's growth or health. Many hours I spent boiling down the sap for just a few ounces of syrup, but the sweetness was well worth the work and effort.

We would never cut down a healthy birch tree, but when one was damaged in a storm, we would utilize so much of it that nothing went to waste. Besides the containers and canoes we would make from the bark, we would collect the inner bark. Dried in the sun, the inner bark can be ground into flour or added directly to stews. The inner bark has a unique taste that is delicious when added with other flours or used alone in the form of ash cakes. The twigs can be steeped in hot water to make a savory tea. For stronger teas, steep longer with hotter water. Boiling removes much of the food value.

Medicinal   I remember a time when I had poison ivy all up my arms, and on my neck and chest. I tried all the old standby medications, starting with calamine lotion, then jewelweed, then finally tannic acid made from boiling acorns. Finally, out of desperation, I asked Stalking Wolf for help, embarrassed that none of the medications I tried worked, feeling a bit of a young failure as an herbalist. He boiled up the twigs of the birch into a strong tea, let it cool slightly, then applied it to my arms and chest, repeating the process twice after it dried. Again he applied the slightly warmed tea at the end of the day. I remember vividly how soothing the tea was to the open sores, almost immediately removing the itch and swelling. He explained that some cases of poison ivy simply will not respond to the regular types of medications and a more specific medication, such as the strong birch tea, is needed for that ailment. I learned quickly that birch can work when others fail and vice versa, depending on the conditions and ailments.

The young leaves used fresh and the supple bark of twigs are the main medicinal parts of the birch. I have gently tried to dry and store the young birch leaves for wintertime use, but with very limited success. The drying removes most of the medicinal properties. I have stored tea made from the leaves in a refrigerator for nearly a month, retaining better than half of the medicinal properties. It is far better to use fresh. The young bark also loses much of its medicinal properties when stored. Fresh bark from the winter tree can be used quite effectively if gathered from lower branches during warm winter days. There are many ways to unlock the healing powers of birch. Each contains its own ritual and strength of medication depending on the illness one uses it for.

A tea made from the leaves produces a diuretic effect. Make the tea by adding a palmful of fresh, young leaves to boiling water. Remove immediately from heat source and let steep for five to ten minutes depending on the severity of the malady. A tea made by this method can also be used as a skin wash for mild skin maladies such as poison ivy, bee stings, and other rashes. A stronger tea medication can be made by boiling the succulent bark and leaves for two to seven minutes. This strong tea can be used as a mild sedative which induces a good night's sleep and a calming effect on the body during times of stress. This same tea boiled for ten minutes can be used as a skin wash or bath additive for severe skin problems and even acne. As an adolescent, I found that the strong birch bark tea was more effective for skin blemishes than the medications sold over the counter at drug stores. Some students with severe acne problems have found it more effective than prescription acne medications.

To make either the mild leaf tea or the stronger bark and leaf tea, use a small palmful of the herb or bark per cup of water. For really strong teas, use double the amount of herb or bark to one cup of water. Apply this stronger solution to severe skin problems three times a day. During times of stress, drink one-half cup of strong tea per day as a sedative.

Black Alder (*Alnus glutinosa*)

Description   The black alder is a tree of damp soils and meadow edges. It is a beautifully straight tree, growing to heights of fifty feet, sometimes more. Its leaves are quite wide, double-toothed with blunt ends, reaching lengths from two to five inches. The young leaves and twigs are quite sticky, especially in spring, when they produce a gummy substance. The tree flowers in mid-spring and its fruits resemble small pinecones, called catkins, on elegant, slender stalks. The trunk of the tree is dark with deeply scarred rings sometimes found close or actually growing together on the older bark. Black alder is found in the northeastern United States, west to Illinois, and south to Delaware.

Personality   On the far, northwestern edge of the Pine Barrens, where the pines blend into the northern deciduous forests, I met my first black alder, but I can't say that my first experience was a pleasant one. There it stood at the edge of a meadow that was once part of an old homestead probably back before the Revolutionary War. I was quite sick to my stomach, a combination of things causing the queasy feeling. Too many green apples, their ripeness questionable, and the very long trek over a number of days put me on the edge of gastrointestinal distress, producing weakness, nausea, and sweats.

Stalking Wolf took a small strip of the tree's bark, which he boiled in a small wooden bowl. After steeping it in the hot water for about five minutes, he gave it to me to drink. I felt as if I couldn't put anything in my stomach, but dutifully, I drank all of the tea. Almost immediately I began to vomit, and even though it only lasted a few minutes, I had thrown up to a point where there were still stomach spasms and nothing left in my stomach. But I began to feel better, far better than I had all day. In a little over an hour I was back on my feet and working up to capacity.

Our camp was not far from this beautiful tree that looked so out of place on the edge of the meadow, yet I found myself giving it a wide berth all day long. It had quite a mystical air about it which intrigued me, but I still had a healthy respect for what it could do to the digestive system. My whole outlook on the tree changed later that day when Rick cut himself on some reed grass, and the cut would not stop bleeding. Grandfather took from his bag a little pouch of powder and sprinkled it across the wound. Like magic the bleeding stopped. A few hours later the wound had scabbed over and Rick was back to work. Curiously, I asked Grandfather what the powder

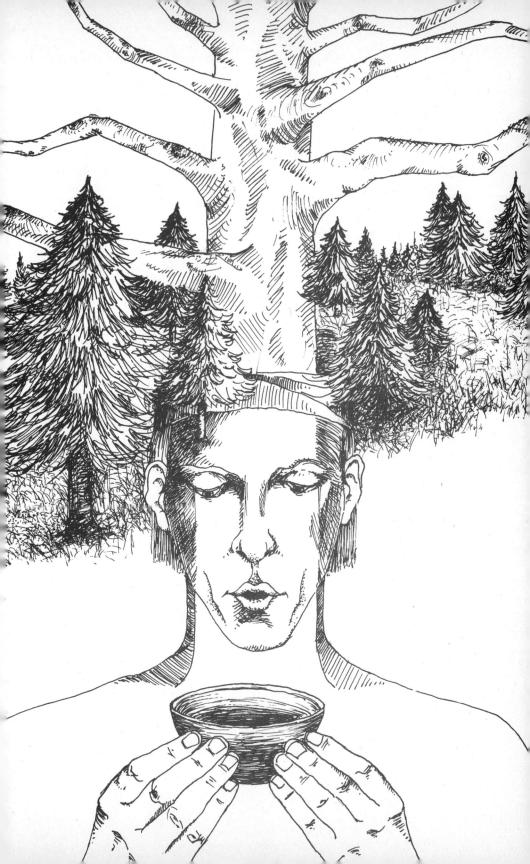

was, and he coyly answered that it was from the same tree bark that had made me vomit.

Grandfather, instinctively aware of my subsequent avoidance of the big tree and noting the shock on my face when he said that the tree had produced both medications, began to teach me of the way any given plant could produce any number of medications depending on the preparations and the time of gathering. The wisdom found in the medicine of that old alder tree was the beginning of my understanding how intricate the medicinal plant world can be. He went on to explain that the fresh bark would produce the vomiting but that dried bark produced other healing results. The vomiting that was produced by the bark was a necessary medication, used in clearing out my stomach and getting me back on my feet. Medication does not have to produce soothing or immediate healing results alone. Some other medications produce good results but are first experienced with a certain distaste or uneasiness.

I've grown to love the black alder, not only as a powerful medicinal healer, but for its grace, form, and elegance in growth. The huge, old black alder at the edge of that little meadow taught me so much. It is still there and growing fine today. So many times I have come back to it for medicine for the body or spirit. Each time I gaze upon its lofty branches, many of them now gnarled by the passing years, I am transported back to the many times we camped near it. I still have a vivid picture of it, growing tall and alone, away from the edge of the nearby forests, standing as if in defiance to time and man's encroachment, at its feet a sea of thick morning meadow mist that causes it to stand out in bold relief from everything else. One can't help but gaze on it and feel its power, its mystery, and its connection to the healing forces of the Earth.

Medicinal   Fresh alder bark, when brewed into a mild tea, will cause vomiting. If vomiting does not occur within a few moments after drinking the tea, make a new batch of stronger tea. A tea made from the dried bark makes a good mouthwash for sore throats, toothaches, or other mouth irritations. A strong tea made from the bark is good for applying to moderate skin irritations, poison ivy, and bee stings. Powdered bark and leaves make a good internal astringent and aid for digestion. Powdered bark also makes a good hemostatic for external hemorrhaging. Mild tea will make a good toothpaste, which not only cleans teeth well, but helps abscessed and decaying teeth.

To prepare the dosages, boil a small palmful of dried bark and leaves in a little over a cup of water. Boil for two to three minutes and let sit for two minutes. Dosage for internal use is one-quarter cup in the morning, and one-quarter cup in the evening. It is best to use young leaves and bark for drying. Collect the bark and leaves in the late spring and early summer. Shred the bark and the leaves and allow to dry slowly in the sun. Grind to a powder and store in a glass or earthenware container in a cool, dry place. Bark collecting in the winter should be done on warm days, using the lower branches. The fresh bark, used to induce vomiting, should be a very small palmful added to one-half to one cup of water. Boil for two minutes, let steep for two minutes.

Boneset (*Eupatorium perfoliatum*)

Description Boneset is a beautiful plant which, to the untrained eye, will look similar to angelica and water hemlock. While white cloudlike flowers suspended on spindly stalks do indeed closely resemble angelica, the flower clusters are farther apart. The plant is generally hairy in texture, the leaves are wrinkled and usually joined at the base, especially the older leaves. The young leaves tend not to be joined. Boneset thrives in low grounds near water, usually in thickets and flowers from mid-summer to mid-fall. It is found in low ground and wet lands from the eastern coastal states from Canada, south to Florida, and west to Texas.

Personality These hazy white flowers with their hairy stems and leaves were always intriguing to me. When you gaze upon the boneset, you can't help but feel its power, knowing instinctively by the way that the leaves grow together that is has tremendous healing and rejuvenating properties. Stalking Wolf always held this plant in the utmost reverence. Near the little swamp area by the Good Medicine Cabin, there was a small patch of these little healers. I would find him there often, talking to them or offering them tobacco, almost like an ancient gardener tending his fields. I knew the boneset well long before I ever tasted its medicinal values.

It was years after our meeting that I felt its powers heal me in such a quick and loving way. By accident or design, I had broken my hand quite badly, and the doctor told me that I would be wearing a cast from six to eight weeks. This news would have been upsetting at any time of the year, but with the oncoming summer, I could see myself sitting out of so many activities, especially those of the water. I told Grandfather of my plight, and he said that he would take care of my malady much faster than the six weeks dictated by the doctor. We went to the boneset patch and made an offering. He pointed to the new little leaves at the top of the plant and asked me to observe how they had grown separately, whereas the lower leaves had grown together as one. That, he said, is what the boneset would do for my broken bones. Though I can't substantiate it medically or with any subsequent scientific investigation, my cast was cut from my hand in two weeks and I had full mobility within the next week.

I drank a tea made from the larger leaves twice a day for the first week, the second week only one-half cup twice a day. Almost immediately, I could feel a difference in the broken area of my hand, a certain tingling feeling as if the knitting process had sped up con-

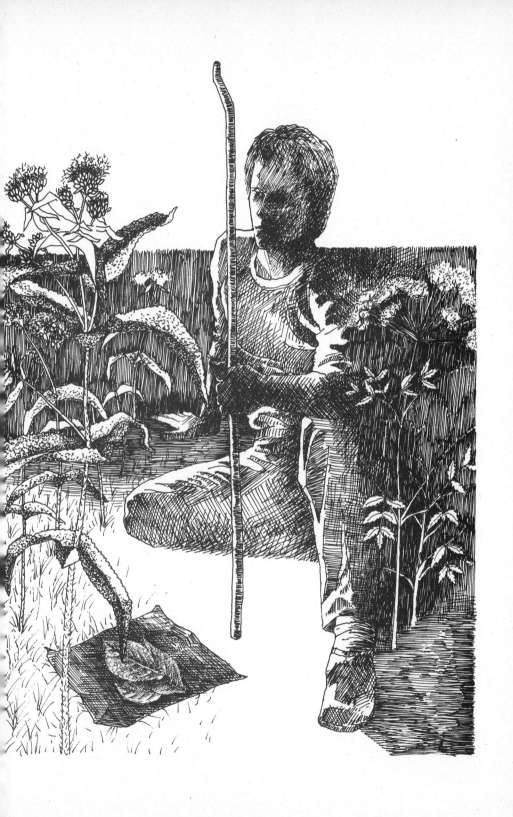

siderably. Even the pain died away quickly and the swelling went down overnight. I have used boneset for every broken bone I have ever had except one. All the broken bones healed in one-half to one-quarter the time anticipated except for the broken bone I used no medication on. That bone took two extra weeks to heal, although it was not a bad break. Needless to say, the doctors were shocked at the rate the bones mended, none of them believing me about the boneset tea, proclaiming it an old wives' tale or Indian lore.

I have even found boneset to work on swollen joints and stiffness, giving a little relief to people suffering from arthritis and rheumatism. I continue to use boneset on myself and many of my students with a great deal of success. A mixture of one-half cup of boneset tea and one-half cup of catnip tea relaxes sore muscles, even strained muscles, with phenomenal results. Some of my students who are also professional movement and massage therapists use this mixture with their patients. When the patients drink the tea one hour before massage, the therapists find them more responsive to the therapy, and the patients also feel the greater heightened effects of the massage.

Some of the old and wise folks I meet on my travels use boneset as a base medication to mix with other medications. Many of the oldest folks I know drink a cup of boneset tea a day and suffer no effects of arthritis or rheumatism. In many parts of this country, it is considered a tonic against aging or for keeping energy up, colds away, and the body moving freely. I know when I have been in winter survival class situations where I am exposed to the threat of colds and flu, I hardly ever got a cold those years that I used the boneset tea on a daily basis. I find that it also seems to improve my circulation, especially to the hands and feet. Those years that I have forgotten to put up the dried herbs for winter use, I have suffered innumerable colds, cold feet, and numerous other winter-related aches and pains.

In all the years I knew Grandfather, I have never seen him sick, not even with a common cold. We, on the other hand, were always exposed to germs and constantly bringing our colds, flu, and fevers back into the woods with us. Whenever Grandfather heard the first sniffle or felt our heads for the first sign of fever, out came the boneset. It was remarkable how it gave us almost instant relief, sometimes throwing off the cold immediately. It continuously astounded our parents and doctors how quickly we could throw off maladies that would put other people out for a week or more. We rarely had a cold or flu longer than three days. Those times we were not so fortunate to find Grandfather during these periods, we held onto colds just as long as everyone else. We were surprised to find out that the same tea that healed my bones was the same tea that killed our colds so effectively. We understood fully why Grandfather so cherished his little patch of boneset and why he carried it around in his healing bag as one of his base healing herbs.

Medicinal There are very few herbal books that proclaim the bone-healing properties of boneset, probably because there is no known scientific proof of these bone-healing properties. I use my own personal experience and the results on other people as proof positive of these and many of the other ancient herbal claims of the potency of this herb. A mild tea made by steeping the fresh or dried perfoliated, joined leaves for fifteen to thirty minutes in hot water makes an excellent bone and joint remedy. Grandfather would use a palmful of fresh or dried leaves to two cups of water.

The effects of the boneset teas depend largely on how they are taken and the preparation and strength of the teas. A cold tea made from steeping a small palmful of dried or fresh leaves in one cup of water for twenty to thirty minutes has a mild, laxative effect and makes a good digestive tonic. A warm tea made essentially the same way, but steeped from thirty to thirty-five minutes, is a great remedy for colds, flu, fever, and for controlling night sweats. A strong tea prepared the same way but taken hot can induce vomiting and has strong laxative properties. The cooling properties of the herb that help fight fever and control night sweats are called refrigerants, and are best taken warm.

I have found that a strong tea made from steeping the dried or green leaves for thirty to forty minutes and mixed with an equal dose of mild mint tea is very effective for breaking up the common cold. As a cold or flu preventative, I steep the fresh or dried leaves in cold water for six to twelve hours, and take a cold quarter cup twice a day. This cold steeping retains much of the vitamin C content of the herb. Leaves can be used fresh or dried, the fresh leaves producing the best results, especially where the vitamin C is needed. The upper unjoined leaves are good for colds, fevers, flu, night sweats, and digestion, whereas the mature joined leaves are great for bone and joint ailments, to induce vomiting, and for laxative properties.

Gather the herb in late spring to mid-summer, especially before it flowers, as many of the properties are dispersed into the flowering energy requirements. I prefer to dry the leaves slowly out of direct sunlight, allowing three days for them to become totally dry. I then lightly break up the leaves until they have a tobacco-like consistency. I store these in loosely woven cotton bags hung from the rafters of a cool, dry place. I never make bags larger than six to eight ounces. One of the best ways I store this herb tea is in cheesecloth bags that hold about a teaspoonful of herb so that it can be readily mixed in hot water the same way you would use a tea bag. This way the tea is quickly available as a daily tonic against common colds and other winter ailments.

Bulrush (*Scirpus validus*)

Description   The bulrush grows in dense stands, and is dark green in color. It loves the mud and the shallows of fresh or brackish water. The stems of these plants are very smooth and round, lack leaves, and have pithy centers. The tops of these elegant stems have clusters of coarse deep brown, flower spikes. They bloom from mid-spring to early fall and are found throughout the tropical United States, but may extend north to Delaware and southern New Jersey.

Personality   Some of my fondest memories are from the bulrush swamps along our bays and in various parts of the Pine Barrens. As children, we found these areas to be mysterious, full of wildlife, crammed with adventure and excitement. For hours on hot summer days, despite the mosquitoes and biting flys, we would wander these swamps trying to unlock their secrets. Because of the thick surrounding mudbanks and the near impenetrable domain of these areas, we knew that we were probably the only ones ever to fully explore these areas. The thought of these uncharted areas made us feel like explorers, possibly discovering at any turn a new plant or animal, never before discovered.

One of our favorite bulrush swamp adventures usually began in mid-spring and lasted right through the summer and into the fall. We would find piles of dead wood and other driftwood along the swamp's edge and begin to create an island in the center of a huge bulrush swamp. We usually piled dead vegetation on top of the driftwood making a huge nestlike affair. We then put up walls around portions of the island, creating a blind or a few blinds depending on the size of the island. We would then take sand, mud, and gravel and make a raised fire-pit area, finishing off the island paradise with a thatch hut. We would spend days, sometimes weeks, on our little island, literally living off the surrounding landscape and watching the wildlife, who began to know us and recognize us as friends.

It was on one of these little islands that we learned of the edibility of the bulrush. We were making bulrush candles by soaking them in hot rendered fat, allowing the pithy centers to soak all the way up the stem. After soaking we could prop them up in a wood dish and light them; some of them would burn like a candle for two or more hours. As we sat there, one of the local muskrats came to the edge of our island to feed. He had a huge bulrush root and was nibbling on the succulent rootlettes rather contentedly, which caused me to promptly ask Grandfather if we could eat any part of the bulrush.

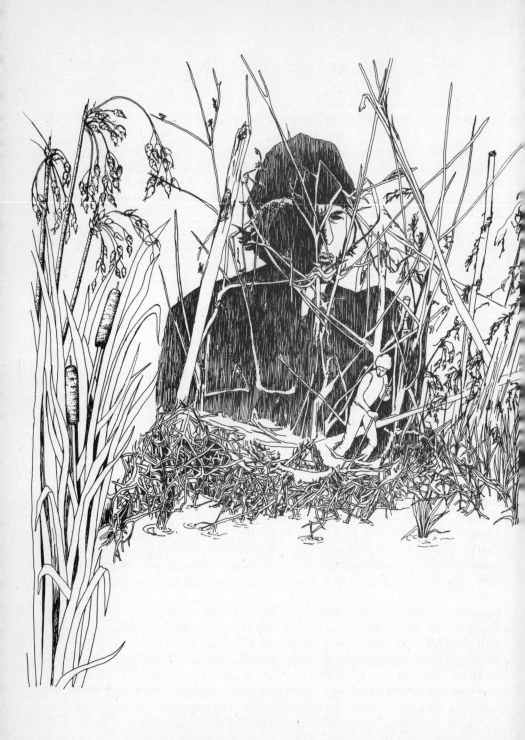

I knew that we could not eat everything that an animal could eat. Many of the things eaten by the animal world are poisonous to humans, but for some reason, the rootlettes being eaten by the muskrat looked rather edible to me.

Grandfather began to unfold all the marvelous edible parts of this tremendous plant brother that we knew so well. We had no idea that we were surrounded by one of the most delicious wild edibles in existence. Not only did the bulrushes provide homes, cover, and food for a wide variety of animals, but it also gave us a cornucopia of food, not to mention the tremendous excitement and adventures we had among their protection. I will never forget that first sweet, succulent taste of bulrush shoots. We dug down into the muddy soil a few inches and pulled up one of the roots. Cooled by the depths of the muddy soil, it was a refreshing treat on a hot summer day. Even in the winter, parts of the roots are edible, and I can't help but feel the promise of summer in every winter bite.

I have a special place in my heart for the bulrush people. So many times they have saved my life and made my survival camps so much easier. Wrapped together they make my baskets, clothing, and blankets. So many times I have slept in bulrush blankets in bitter cold and snow, warm and content, never feeling the elements. Bound together in loglike masses, then tied into a canoe shape, they have made my boats, which have carried me down rivers, across bays, and even challenged the ocean's surf. They are more than food and adventure, they are lasting friends and the very essence of good survival living.

Food The young, tender shoots of the plant are excellent eaten raw, as are the tender cores of the older shoots' bases. There is a refreshing sweetness to the plant, a taste that reminds one of summertime. One can't help but feel the essence of the primal ooze that cradles the roots, experiencing a kinship with the very muck they grow in. The young shoots and inner cores of the older shoots are also excellent cooked. I boil them briefly or steam them to produce a delicious crispy vegetable, much like the bamboo shoots found in Chinese food. The pollen as well as the ground seeds can be dried thoroughly and made into a delicious flour that can be used for a nutritious bread or as a soup thickener. The rootstock tips can be roasted for four hours then eaten much like the potato. The roasted rootstock can also be dried and ground into flour and added half and half to the seed flour or used alone. The breads produced from the rootstock flour are not as sweet as the breads produced by the ground seeds and pollen, but to me they have a wilder and more exotic taste.

Ash cakes made by combining 50 percent bulrush rootstock flour with acorn flour are very rich and nutritious. My first taste of the bulrush-acorn ash cake came during a long trek when we made a bagful of ash cakes to eat along our way. The nourishment that we received kept us going for quite some time, giving us energy and resistance to the cold, without really sitting down and having a full meal. A counterpart to these ash cakes would be the cowboy hardtack which has been mentioned throughout literature. The bulrush is a plant of many seasons, available to us at any time of the year. In the spring, I collect the new shoots and find them a great trailside nibble. In summer, I collect the pollen and dry it for future use. In fall, I collect the seeds, dry them and store them throughout the winter months. From late fall through early spring, the rootstocks are always available and at the peak of their nutrition. Truly, this is an all-around survival plant.

Medicinal   The medicinal value of the bulrush has long since been forgotten. I remember a time I had gotten a puncture wound that quickly grew infected and full of pus. Stalking Wolf took the hard rootstock, poulticed it using tannic acid made from acorn boilings, and applied the paste to the wound. Within a few hours, the wound began to drain and clear up the infection. I have also used the same poultice on severe bee stings, poison ivy blisters, and other skin irritations, with fantastic results.

Bunchberry (*Cornus canadensis*)

Description   At first glance, the flowering bunchberry looks like a small, elegant umbrella with the leaves in whirls of six. The large flower portion is not actually one flower, as indicated at a distance, but a cluster of tiny flowers surrounded by four petallike bracts. Berries are bright red and tightly clustered, each cluster two to eight inches long. Flowers blossom in the late spring to early summer, and the fruits appear from late summer to mid-fall. Bunchberry loves the cold woods and mountain slopes, growing in Canada and the adjacent United States, south to northern West Virginia, via mountain slopes.

Personality   I remember the bunchberry vividly because I learned a tremendous lesson when I first encountered it. Grandfather and I had taken a long trip to the hills of northern New Jersey, and I came across a small patch of these pretty little plants growing on a slope of the deeper section of the forest. Their bright red berries stood out from the mosaic of forest litter, in bold relief from all the greenery that surrounded it. I was intrigued by the berries and the way they were clustered upon the umbrella of leaves. There seemed to be an air of mystery about them, as if they shouldn't really be there, possibly planted by some exotic herbalist to fool amateur naturalists like me. I lay for a long time studying these little plants, imagining that they must be nature's answer to a Christmas-like decoration, except earlier in the season. Some of the plants had whitish berries that were immature, while just a few others had beautiful white flowers, so delicate that I could hardly feel them when I touched their petals.

Grandfather had a good way of teaching us about plants. He gently plucked a few berries and handed them to me to eat. It wasn't enough to just eat the berries, we had to enjoy them to the fullest. For years I had been sampling plants and making them part of my diet, savoring their tastes, their essence, and their spirits to a point where I knew the plant well. The bunchberry presented a culinary problem in many ways; it was almost tasteless, a little bland at best, with no real scent or texture.

This little plant taught us to do more than just taste something. Every day, people are cramming down all sorts of foods and never really tasting them. They do the same with water, wine, and many other beverages. The little bunchberry is a plant that needs far more attention then most herbalists give it. One must probe deeper than the taste senses to discover its delicious essence. The bunchberries

73

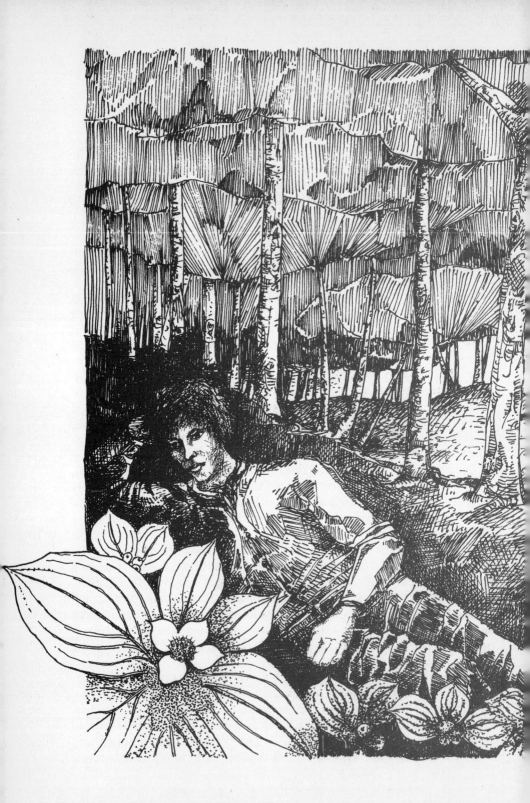

have to be savored slowly to capture their delicate taste fully. In them, one can find a faint sweetness and a unique flavor. We tend to get so used to foods with powerful tastes that we miss the taste of many of the delicate culinary plants. Our bunchberry lesson taught us to slow down and savor food completely. It taught us about tastes that normally go unnoticed by most people, those same people that ignorantly call the plant bland or insipid.

Everything we do in society seems to be pushed to the sensory limits. We take notice of loud stereos, but fail to hear the music of insect wings; we need strong perfumes, but fail to catch the fragrance of some of the tiny delicate wildflowers; we need grand natural vistas to stimulate our awe in Creation, but miss the tiny crystalline pebbles at our feet or the tapestry of animal tracks. The bunchberry is a grand teacher of the sublime, scents so delicate, tastes so subtle, a plant that must be savored slowly to be understood.

Food The bunchberry can be eaten raw as a trailside nibble. As stated earlier, many people find the bunchberry tasteless; but if one slows down long enough, he will find they have a delicate taste beyond description, a sweetness of the faintest essence. The bunchberry, despite its lack of powerful taste, packs good nutritional value. Be careful not to eat the unripened berries, as they may cause stomach upset in some people.

The berries can be added to ash cakes, cooked into stews, or lightly boiled into a cranberrylike sauce. One of my favorite recipes is to take about four cups of berries, two cups of water, and a cup of honey, mix together and boil until a thick sauce consistency is acquired. Use the sauce much as you would cranberry sauce, either added as a topping to other foods or eaten alone. The sauce is also great on ash cakes or, if you are at home, on pancakes.

Medicinal I have used the bunchberry successfully in the treatment of small localized first- and second-degree burns. The berries can be crushed or lightly chewed, and pressed over the burn like a poultice. A more effective medication can be had by boiling a cupful of berries in one-half cup of tannic water. I have also used the tannic/bunchberry poultice for effective relief of itching due to poison ivy, bee stings, and other skin maladies.

The first time I ever used bunchberry as a medication occurred when my hand was burned by scalding water during a hike. Grandfather boiled up some tannic/bunchberry water, cooled it, then applied the cooling poultice to the burn. It felt so soothing, penetrating deep under the burn while relieving the pain. The burn poultice was then washed off after one-half hour. I finished the hike without any discomfort from the burn, which also did not blister as badly as it should have.

Burdock (*Arctium lappa*)

Description The burdock loves waste ground and disturbed soils. They are biennial plants that produce large, rough basal leaves the first year, and bushy flower stalks the second. The flowers are deep purple and give way to the classic thistlelike burr in the fall. It flowers in late summer and early fall. It is found throughout the northeastern United States and up into Canada.

Personality The burdock plant always conjures up thoughts of the prehistoric. It has oversized leaves that could easily hide a young boy. As a child, I spent hours sitting in burdock thickets, awaiting animals. Hidden in these huge leaves, I felt as if I was living at a time when dinosaurs roamed; at other times, I imagined I was a small insect living in someone's lawn. The burdock thickets have always been a place of mystery. The animal trails and runs form vast roadways, more intricate than any manmade roadway system. In these thickets, one feels part of the Earth, cradled in the lush greenery, feeling the rich loamy dampness underneath. The source of wonder never ends. Birds flit in and out of dark green hollows while animals travel the roadway networks. Myriads of insects, grubs, toads, and smaller plants make up the whole mystical minijungle. The streams are always intriguing, always full of adventure, and filled with exciting new discoveries at every dark bend in the trail.

Today I teach my classes on an old farm. All the hedgerows contain huge burdock thickets that offer a sense of childlike reprieve from the rigors of my teaching. On hot summer days, I go into the thickets to escape the sun, finding a place of seclusion that contains its own unique atmosphere, like a thick rain forest or jungle. In this green maze of tunnels and caves, one succumbs to a feeling of deep relaxation and of certain peace, as if in a cool, damp, small temple, removed from the sun and pressures of daily life. Even today as I lay back in the thickets, I am transported back in time and memory to my childhood and my unending fascination with the burdock plants. They are still as exciting and mysterious today as they were twenty some years ago, but now they even hold more peace and relaxation.

Rick and I played in burdock thickets at all times of the year. One of my favorite times was when the plants were in bloom, their deep purple lended easily to the exotic, junglelike feel. The flowerheads were always full of wonder and beauty, so unusual, as if belonging to another time and place. In the winter, the burdock skeletons afford new adventures. For hours, Rick and I used to play a

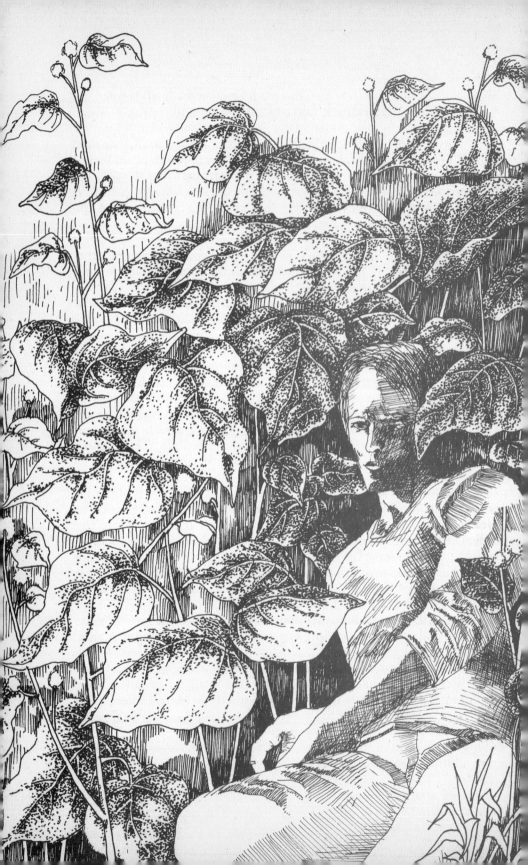

game of scout and cavalry, stalking each other with burr bombs, always ending in all-out wars. I remember the many hours I spent
having burrs pulled from my hair, and I know I have done my share
in spreading new burdock seeds.

My intrigue with the burdock is not all on a spiritual level, for
its survival and medicinal uses are almost endless. It began after one
of those endless burdock wars. Rick and I were both hot and sweaty,
even though the cold winds and low temperatures of that late autumn
day would normally make us quite cold. We were covered with burrs
and mud, and we smelled from cutting the sinew from an old dead
animal. We were forced to take a cold bath in a stream, despite the
fact that young boys hardly ever notice when they get a little rank.

After the cold stream, I slipped into a warm set of clothes, but
the shirt had no buttons. Rick walked up to me as I attempted to sew
my shirt together with a bone awl and some of the fresh and ripe
sinew. He placed a burr on the corner of my shirt and closed the open
half over it; it held together fast. We laughed at his comment about
survival Velcro, but it worked remarkably well. For years I have used
the simple burr to fasten together clothing, sleeping bags, blankets,
and other articles of clothing in need of fast repair. Sometimes I
wonder if the inventors of Velcro have ever spent time in a burdock
patch, thus formulating their ideas.

Burdock goes beyond the uses as a binder of clothing, as it also
feeds us, medicates us, and is a tremendous survival plant for all
times of the year. Burdock leaves have wrapped my fish and other
foods during their pit cooking. The leaves have shingled the roofs of
my temporary summer survival shelters and have also been used as
quick clothing. The burrs stick together and make fine mats or tinder
holders. The skeletons make good fire drills, both hand and bow
methods. The burdock is always there, not only to relax and comfort
me but to feed me and otherwise care for me when the going gets
rough.

Food   I remember well the first taste of burdock root. It was
a bitter cold winter day and we had traveled overnight to reach our
camp location, without food or rest. We were thoroughly exhausted
and very cold. Grandfather sat down next to a burdock skeleton and
made a fire using the straight stalk of the plant. Immediately we had
that fire, thanks to the quick-starting stem and smaller burdock
branches we used as kindling. He then built a few smaller fires on
top of some first-year leaf clusters of our burdock brothers. Within a
half hour, he removed the fire from the now-thawed ground and dug

the root of the plant. We melted some snow and boiled the peeled roots in water for a little over one-half hour, then changed the water and boiled again until they were tender. I guess it was the carbohydrates found in the roots that energized us, but I felt like a new man after that meal. It gave us more than enough strength to build our survival camp and do our chores before needing to rest or eat again.

Burdock is one of my favorite edibles, but the taste usually has to be acquired because it can be a little bitter and wild tasting. The young, succulent leaves can be added fresh to salads, blending in their rather unique taste to brighten any salad. I also use the young leaves as a cooked herb, boiling them in four changes of water for a total of one-half hour of slow boiling. This frequency of water changing removes much of the bitter taste and makes them tender. I eat my burdock leaves raw as a trailside nibble when I am on long excursions, but the taste must be slowly acquired. I do not recommend eating large quantities of the young leaves, for they can cause upset stomachs, and sometimes even cramps or diarrhea.

The roots of the first-year plants can be dug from the ground, peeled of their bitter inedible rind and boiled for one-half hour, using two or three changes of water. Rootstalks used in the fall and winter are tough and a little bitter as compared to the early summer roots. I save any left-over cooked roots, dry them in the sun, and store them to be ground up and used later as a soup or stew thickener. The young leafstalks and flowerstalks can be peeled off the green rind, revealing a soft white inner core which can be eaten raw, added to salads, or cooked the same way as the roots. They can be cooked, dried, and stored the same way we did with the left-over rootstocks.

Medicinal   I came upon one of the medicinal uses of the burdock leaf the same way I came upon the survival use of the burr: by accident. I had a bad case of poison ivy on my forearm and it itched incessantly. I got fed up with the external itching and grabbed a burdock leaf, sensing that it might be used the same way a plantain plant could be used. I rubbed the leaf over the affected area quite briskly, and within minutes the pain and itch were gone. Since then I have applied the raw leaf to all sorts of skin rashes, bites, and even boils with the same remarkable results. To prepare it as a poultice for a bee sting, chew a section of leaf and apply it, for the best quick emergency results.

For mild skin problems, soak the fresh or dried leaves or roots in cold water for six to eight hours. This mild astringent can also be used effectively for minor open wounds as a mild antiseptic. Roots of the second-year plant are best for medicinal uses and should be collected in early spring or fall. The root and leaves can be dried slowly in the sun, broken up to the consistency of tobacco, and stored in a glass or earthenware container. The rind of the root and leafstalk should not be removed as these have many of the medicinal properties needed for skin problems. A stronger skin medication can be made from simmering the root or leaves for fifteen minutes, thirty minutes for more strength. The usual recipe is a handful of fresh leaves or root to three cups of water, or a palmful of dried root or leaves to one cup of water.

The tea made from the root or leaves is great for stomach ailments. With most people, it can be used as an effective laxative, but in some cases, it may cause diarrhea. The tea is very soothing to the stomach and bowels; it also induces mild sweating and has diuretic properties. Many old-timers use the tea as a maintenance drink when they find themselves coming down with a common cold or other ailment. I have found it very useful in getting my system back in order after an intestinal flu. The usual dosage is one-half cup twice a day. It is good to start off with a weak tea made from soaking a small palmful of root or leaf in a cup of water for four hours; increase soaking up to eight hours for stronger tea. I find the latter good for relieving stomach cramps. A strong tea also can be made by simmering root or leaves in water for ten minutes. Usual dosage is a small palmful of plant parts to a cup of water. Since allergic reactions to any substance are always a possibility, I do caution first-time users to go easy on the internal medicinal teas.

Catnip (*Nepeta cataria*)

Description   Catnip loves disturbed soils, waste grounds, and roadsides. It flowers from late spring to early fall. The flowers are absolutely gorgeous, found at the end of the stems in thick clusters, soft violet to white in color, with purplish spots. The leaves are arrowhead shaped, very jagged, and gray-green with a frosting of white downy exteriors. Catnip has a mild minty odor. It is found throughout the United States and beyond.

Personality   There is a certain alluring quality about catnip. It is not an exotic or unique plant in overall appearance, but rather benign. It blends easily into any plantscape, drawing no attention to itself, as is the case with so many powerful herbs. One has to look close and low in the overall scheme of things to even begin to understand this little mint plant and its aura of surrounding power. This ability to blend with the landscape and its total power are part of the charisma this little plant has over me. It's like a beautiful lesson in philosophy, stating in its leaves the essence of quiet power: subtle and plain on the outside, dynamically powerful inwardly.

When the plant is growing out in bold relief from the surrounding vegetation, it cannot help but captivate one. Even though it is very plain at first glance, those who look closer will be thoroughly delighted. It seems to appear as a fountain of green, embellished with a frosty white hue, as if pumped from the Earth like some surrealistic frothing green water. The faint scent cast from the delicate flowers is almost intoxicating. It brings to mind the feel of warm summer days, of peace and tranquillity, whenever one catches the elusive fragrance.

Until I was introduced to catnip by Grandfather, I only gave it mild attention. To my young mind, there were so many other more exotic and interesting plants to explore and savor. I hardly gave it any thought, other than when it was in bloom, for the flowers were always intriguing. It was during the catnip blossom time that I was introduced to catnip on a more intimate level, and I began to see its inner beauty. It wasn't until I learned to look beyond the physical and into the core that I learned what true beauty is.

Grandfather was asked to come to the house of an old friend who needed his help. Apparently, the friend was suffering from anxiety as a result of financial problems concerning his little farm. I knew from past experience that Grandfather was a good friend to many of

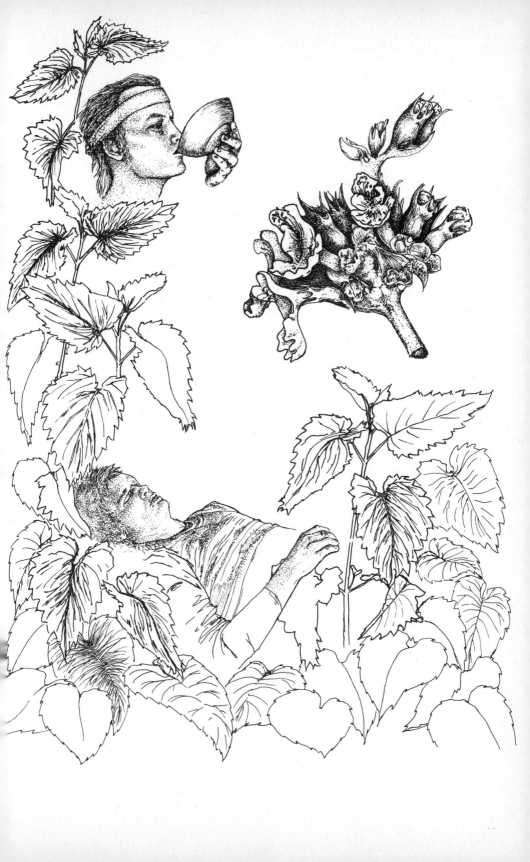

the old-timers of the area, but this was the first time I ever saw him work as a herbal doctor. Listening to the two men talk, I realized what an influence he had on the people of the area, especially on a medicinal level. I never realized that he had been seeing many of the people as patients for years, and this old man was no exception.

I became involved with catnip as a result of this old man and his condition. I realized the importance of Grandfather asking me to come with him, and I was very honored that he wanted me along as his apprentice/assistant. They talked for a while, Grandfather acting much like a psychiatrist but on a deeper level. He had to develop a feeling for the medication that would calm the condition. This talk and inner sense of the patient is very important to the level of medication. Each medication has to be custom-made to fit the patient, unlike the mass medication found in drug stores. Herbal medication is very personal and patient-oriented. Its mixing, collecting, and preparation are so intricate that a chemist or pharmacist might even be surprised.

I was sent out into an old abandoned field on the south side of a small hill, where the catnip would possess the power needed for this medication. I understood that where a plant grew, what stage it was in, and the type of soil were all important in the potency of the plant, so I took great care in selecting the plant that Grandfather wanted. I prayed to the plant first because communication and understanding is an important part of the medication. I then carefully selected a few of the tiny, succulent leaves just beneath the top of the plant. Grandfather asked that I not take the leaves from a blooming plant, as the flowerheads only removed the power from the leaves.

The anxiety of the old man had manifested as insomnia, so Stalking Wolf began to prepare the medication late in the day. First he took the leaves and allowed them to dry in the sun until the end of the day. These were not fully dry but broke easily when he began to prepare them for the tea. Just before the old man went to bed, Grandfather boiled some water, added the semidry leaves, and let the tea steep for about one-half hour, consoling the patient the whole time, assuring him that things would be all right. Grandfather had a tremendous, caring bedside manner. The old man drank the full cup of tea and went to bed.

The next day we were passing the farm when we saw the old man sitting on the porch. Grandfather inquired as to how he had slept and found that he had slept soundly for over ten hours. My heart soared at the thought that I had helped this old man in even some small way. I saw the results of the catnip tea, its soothing qualities, and the way it mellowed the body and spirit. I realized then the power of its sedative qualities and one of its many uses.

Food   Collect the new succulent green leaves throughout the spring, summer, and early fall. Dry the leaves by hanging them in bunches in a cool dry place, and store in a glass or earthenware container for future use. Brew as a soothing tea by steeping in hot water for about ten minutes. A tea also can be made by steeping the fresh green leaves in hot water for fifteen minutes. It can be served hot or cold.

Medicinal   My first medicinal introduction to catnip came during a sweat-lodge ceremony. I was quite dirty, from a hot, dusty hike, to a point where the dirt was caked on my skin. I was also having trouble with an infected hair follicle on my shoulder, due to the rubbing of a strap from a heavy bundle. Grandfather said that a sweat lodge would help clean my pores and get the duct of the hair follicle working again so it could drain. After drinking plenty of water, Grandfather gave me a big mug of very strong catnip tea. He explained that the tea would promote profuse sweating very much like the yarrow, and sweat I did. It felt as if my body had become a waterfall, and I could feel my pores blown wide open. As I exited the sweat lodge, I felt cleaner than I ever had before. The next day, any traces of the abscess and pus buildup were gone. I did, however, find it necessary to drink almost two gallons of water in the next twenty-four hours.

To make a good tea, use the fresh herb made from the new green leaves for a strong tea, the dried herb from the new green leaves for a regular tea. Use one small palmful of broken leaves to about one cup of boiling water. Let the tea steep for ten to twenty minutes depending on the strength of the tea needed. Dosage is one to three cups a day, not to exceed four days. Tea is also good for pain, cramps, and intestinal problems, and has a soothing quality that has a calming effect on most people.

The best leaves to collect are from plants growing in a partially sunny area, preferably with a southeast exposure. Collect leaves before the flowerheads develop. For milder teas, collect the leaves as the flowerhead is developing, or until the seeds are produced. I find that one of the most potent stages of the plant is when it is collected either in early spring or the second blooming of late fall. As an herbalist, I collect the plant beginning in the spring, and ending in the fall when it turns brown. I place the collection in separate containers and label them accordingly so they can fit the needs of the people that come to me.

The general tea dosages are as follows: To induce sweating, one cup of strong tea made by steeping the dried leaves for twenty minutes in hot water. To relieve pain, steep the dried or green leaves in hot water from seven to twelve minutes. To relieve stomach cramps and intestinal disorders, double the dosage of herb to one cup of water and simmer for fifteen minutes; this can be taken hot or cold, depending on the season. For a soothing tea that promotes relaxation, use the tiny leaves which are found below the developing flower-heads and that have been dried in a cool, dry place; allow these leaves to steep for twenty minutes.

Cattail (*Typha spp.*)

Description   This elegant, stately plant, with its swordlike leaves, stems straight and unbranched, and topped with a cylindrical, sausagelike head, is familiar to most people. The cylindrical head starts out as tiny flowers topped with golden secondary pollen spikes which disappear later. As the cattail matures, it turns from green to the familiar brown. Cattails flower in late spring, and is found in shallow water and fresh or brackish marshes throughout the United States and into Canada.

Personality   As a boy, there was nothing like a cattail swamp to conjure up excitement in me. Looking out over any cattail swamp will immediately reveal some of the wonders going on all about these beautiful places. On the various stalks, one can see the red-winged blackbird or hear its song as swallows flit over the greenery. All manner of animal—insect, fish, and fowl—love this area. Because of its protection and the water beneath, it becomes a haven to so much wildlife. Always astir, day and night, with songs of frogs, insects, and birds, it is a lively place to come and sit. For those hearty souls or young adventurous boys, a cattail swamp affords endless exploration and excitement if one doesn't mind getting muddy and wet. To me, the cattail swamps were the most exotic of all the places we used to play. For hours, we would wade or swim in and out of the swamps, stalking animals, watching fish, or just getting involved in the scheme of things. The cattail swamps were like no other place on Earth, and we just couldn't get enough of them.

One of our favorite things to do in the huge cattail swamp we called Muskrat Run was to build a huge raft. Much like Tom Sawyer, we would be free to explore the far reaches of the swamp. As we got older, our rafts became more refined, some actually having fire pits and shelters right onboard. We lived on the rafts and in the swamps for weeks at a time, eating from the cattail, making fires, thatch blankets, and clothing materials. Essentially, we depended on the cattail for everything, including our sense of wonder and enjoyment.

As time passed and we learned more of what the cattail could be used for, we began to experiment and come up with our own ideas. We certainly used the cattail head (punk) soaked in tallow, to burn as a torch and as a smudge to rid the area of mosquitoes, and as an addition to our tinder bundles. We soon discovered what a great insulation the cattail down was, and began to incorporate it into our clothing. One of my favorite things was to get two old blankets and

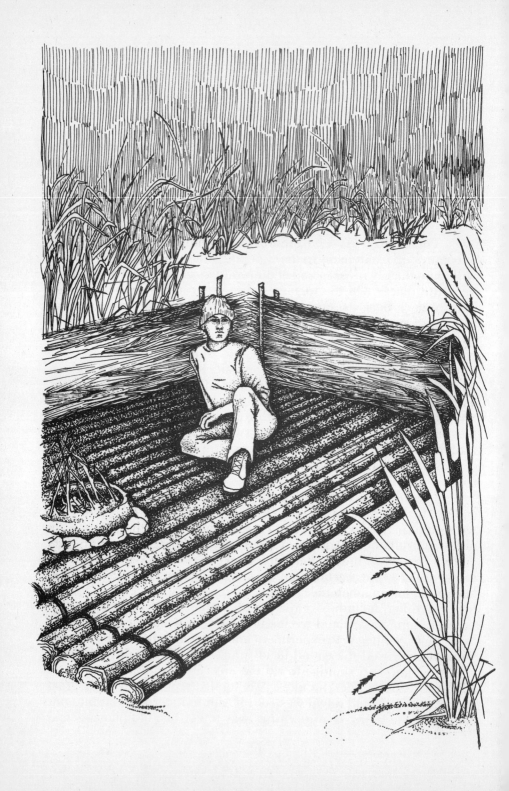

sew them together with an opening at the top. Into the opening we would stuff cattail down until it made a huge pillowlike affair. These we used as sleeping bags through the winter, and they kept us warm and snug in all types of weather. At the end of the season, we would shake out the cattail down, thus reseeding the swamps, and wash our makeshift bags.

We used the cattail for mats, shelter, food, warmth, making fire, making rafts, medication, and so many other things. By the time I was twelve, I knew the cattail quite well and could easily pick out all edible and medicinal parts, but as always, there was still very much to learn. While collecting some pollen for our stews and bread, Grandfather approached and sat watching for a long time. We began to get a little careless with our collection and failed to ask the plants for their help. Grandfather called to us from the bank and we sat down near him to listen to his stories. We knew that we had done something wrong by the tone of his voice and his gestures. He made us realize how important it is not to get careless, no matter how abundant the food plant. That kind of greed, he said, only breeds contempt and a complacency toward the Earth. He went on to explain that things are not always as they seem, for the cattail-pollen we were collecting was not only edible but very sacred to his people. We would dishonor them if we were to continue to be careless with our collection. Every plant is owned by the Creator and the spirit-that-moves-through-all-things, and should be treated with respect. If we treat plants with little respect, soon we treat animals with little respect, and soon the Earth, then finally our fellow humankind. We learned from Grandfather and the cattail swamp to treat all things of the earth, sky, and water with the utmost respect and reverence.

The cattail plant itself held us in awe. Its many medicinal, edible, and survival uses were very intriguing, but the plant itself fascinated us. It was so tall and elegant, growing with its feet in the water, its slender stalk giving way to sword-shaped leaves, and then, finally, to the punk, the cattail itself. It is a gorgeous plant, and when many are growing together, one is inspired by the Creator's work and the marvelous way plants can adapt to most any condition.

Food   The first taste of cattail was one I will always remember. We were playing in the swamp when Grandfather began digging down into the mud and extracted a cattail root. He took it to the stream, gently washed it off, and began to collect the little pearly white, cone-shaped corms growing along its length. He did not take them all but allowed a few to remain, planting the root back in the mud to insure more cattail growth later that spring. We all feasted on the raw corms, so delicious, refreshing, and filling. We sat by the edge of the swamp, watching the pulsating spring activity, feeling the cattail corms drawing us to a closer union with the swamp than we ever felt before.

Cattail has many deliciously edible parts. It is not an acquired taste, as with many of the wild edible plants, and will please even the most finicky. No matter what time of the year you seek out the cattail, there is always something edible and very nutritious. It is one plant the survivalist can depend on, no matter what the situation. When other plants are long gone to seed, and the roots of many others frozen in the earth, the cattail provides easy access to its parts, thus becoming a much needed and appreciated friend.

In the spring, we gather the young succulent shoots, which can be pulled from the rootstock without digging. Once peeled to reveal their tender white core, they can be eaten raw or cooked like a vegetable. I prefer the shootstock crispy, so I steam for only ten minutes. Those who like softer vegetables can boil them up to fifteen minutes. The young shoots can be gathered until they are a little over two feet tall. The green flowerstalks can be removed from their sheaths and can be eaten much like corn on the cob. I find that steaming rather than boiling keeps much of the flavor. If I boil the immature spikes, I leave on the papery sheaths until cooked.

The pollen can be gathered from the yellow pollen spikes in early summer. This pollen can be laid in the sun to dry and be used half-and-half with regular flour or any of the wild edible flours. I use it as a soup or stew thickener and store much of it for winter use, as it is rich in protein. I also use the pollen like a hot cereal, simmering it in water for one-half hour until it grows thick like oatmeal; it is eaten the same way. I find, too, that the pollen is a great additive to pancakes or scrambled eggs.

In late summer, small horn-shaped cones begin to form on the rootstock and remain until the following spring, where they mature into the new shoots. These corms can be eaten raw much like the flour spikes or cooked much the same way. At the base of each of these corms is a starchy base that I like to eat raw, but most people prefer to cook like a potato by either steaming, baking, or boiling.

One of the best parts of cattail is the flour derived from the rootstock. During its dormant months, the rootstocks can be dug from the muck, rinsed clean, and broken up in fresh water. This helps to remove the starchy flour from the fibers of the rootstock. It is best to peel off the outer covering of the rootstock before breaking it up in the water. The flour should be allowed to settle to the bottom of the container, the water poured off, new water poured in, shaken and allowed to settle once again. The process should be repeated one or two more times with any of the remaining fiber or grit being picked out. The pollen must be spread in the sun and allowed to dry slowly. Once thoroughly dried, it can be stored and used the same way as store-bought flour.

One of Grandfather's favorite recipes was to mix one-third root flour with one-third pollen flour and one-third boiled and crushed corm bases. Made into ash cakes, these produced a fine, energy-rich trail bread that would last several days. Cattail flour also makes a good pemmican additive combining one-quarter tallow, one-quarter partially dried and ground berries, one-quarter jerky, and one-quarter cattail pollen or flour. Mixed together to a doughball-like consistency, it adds a better taste to regular blend pemmican.

Medicinal   For a binder to control diarrhea, tea made by adding a small palmful of cattail rootstock flour to one cup of hot water makes an effective remedy. The usual dosage is two cups a day. At the base of each green leaf, there is a sticky substance which is good for use on cuts and abrasions. I find that, in many cases, the substance not only is an effective antiseptic and coagulant, but also has numbing properties. I have used this sticky juice for deadening the pain of toothaches with good results.

The pasty starch of the root has a soothing effect on poison ivy and burns. The boiled and cooled corm bases can be directly applied to boils, bee stings, and other infections to help draw out or drain the infection. I have used a pollen and tallow mixture as a hair conditioner when my hair has been badly damaged by wind, sun, or weather. The boiled leaves of cattail also makes a good external skin wash for rashes and other skin maladies. I use a burning cattail head to fumigate my shelters and generally keep insects away from camp. Once the cattail down is removed from the stalk, the fuzzy stalk can be used as a toothbrush with the flour from the rootstock as a paste.

Chicory (*Cichorium intybus*)

Description   It is an elegant plant with beautiful blue flowers, the rays square-tipped and fringed, sometimes pink or even white in color. They have the mystical habit of closing by late afternoon or when a storm is threatening. The sap is milky, and the basal leaves look very much like a dandelion's. The flowers are stalkless with hardly any leaves, and the whole plant seems to be composed only of these beautiful flowers floating along its stem. The root is white, fleshy, and thick. Chicory is found throughout the United States, inhabiting roadsides, waste places, and disturbed soils.

Personality   My early fascination with plants became manifested with chicory. I was on my way to the river to look for Great Blue Heron tracks when I first encountered this beautiful plant. The rich blue flowers stood out dramatically from the surrounding foliage and captured my sight with their vibrant color. I was further intrigued by this plant on my way back from the river. The skies had become overcast, and now the blue flowers had turned a pale white and were beginning to close up. I thought that they might be dying, but the next day they were open and as blue as ever. A repeat of conditions brought me back to the chicory, and I watched as they turned from deep blue to white then partially closed up. Upon the return of sunny skies at mid-morning, they were again open and reversing the process, not unlike a herbal weatherman. Upon further investigation, I found that the plants closed up every afternoon and did not reopen until the following morning.

I was so fascinated by the chicory flowers that I spent days studying them. I used to lie for hours, watching carefully for any movement or change in the color of the flower. I would watch the weather systems and cloud movement to see what effect they had on the overall plant. At times, I became upset when the flowers finally closed in the afternoon because I knew that my watching was done for the day. To me, they had some strange inner power that was connected to the universe. I desperately wanted to unlock their secret. To make matters worse, the flowers didn't close all at the same time, some closing hours after the rest had gone in for the day. Once in a while, one would stay open for a day or two, defying all the laws, and I searched soil type, growing location and position to find the whys of it all. After quite a few weeks of intense study, I could tell when a storm was coming, what kind of weather was expected, and how long it would last by the way the chicory flowers would close up. To me, they were the weather prophets of the plant world.

Grandfather was very pleased at my dedication to the observation of the chicory. Day after day he would watch me lying or sitting by the plants, talking to them, or taking notes. To him, I must have been exhibiting all the qualities of a future herbalist, but to me, it was a challenge to unlock the secrets of the flowers. After observing for so many days, I instinctively knew that the plant had tremendous power and potential on many levels, even before Grandfather started unlocking its secrets for me. Its edibility and medicinal values were in no way a shock or surprise. Nothing he could have told me about the chicory was beyond belief, for I felt a certain kinship to it, a binding of spirits that can come only from long and intimate contact. I felt as if I had discovered the plant for myself and all the other subsequent information was after the fact.

I had been eating chicory for years before I ever saw the medicinal uses of the plant. Ironically, the first time I saw the power of the plant released was not on a human but on our dog Butch. Butch had an abscess on his lower back, the result of a wound received in one of his fights with a local dog. Our parents couldn't afford to have the dog taken care of by the vet, so, as with all our animals, we had to provide the care. We kept the wound clean, washing it several times a day, but the abscess only continued to get worse.

We wrapped up a bag of tobacco, as a gift to Stalking Wolf, and headed over to his camp. Whenever we approached Grandfather for a healing, we did it in the old way. We would take him a gift, ask for his help, and then allow him to think about it for a while. This protocol was important to the healer so that he knew how much we really needed the healing, and it also gave him time to think about the patient. Knowing the patient, taking the time to know all about him, is an important force in the healing process, unlike the cold, removed attitudes found in doctor-patient relationships today. The more intimately a herbalist knows his patient, the better he can tailor the herbal remedy to fit the patient's exact needs.

Grandfather knew Butch very well, so it wasn't long before he emerged from his shelter and accompanied us back to the house. He looked at the abscess carefully. In a soft, soothing voice, he tried to make Butch calm and receptive. We gathered some fresh chicory leaves and flowers, placed them in a clean cotton cloth, then simmered them in water for about fifteen minutes. We allowed the poultice to cool a bit, then Grandfather placed it directly on the wound, holding it in place for quite a while. The procedure was repeated twice more with fresh herbs. Several hours later, the abscess was reduced, and it didn't seem as sore to Butch anymore. From that day on, there was a bond between Grandfather and Butch, and it wasn't too long afterward that Butch moved out of his doghouse and into Grandfather's shelter.

Food One of my fondest memories of chicory came after an afternoon spent in cold water. Rick and I had floated down a good portion of Cedar Creek. Even though it was late spring, the water was still quite cold, and our five-mile float was interrupted frequently by what we called sun breaks. A sun break was accomplished by pulling our cold, numb bodies from the water and finding a sunny place to warm ourselves. The stream floats, though painful at times, were very necessary at this time of year because they afforded us the best view of the spring birds that inhabited the stream banks. The streams were always a source of new discoveries and beautiful sights, drawing us down their icy waters to the places people could not reach. Many of the smaller streams we explored had probably not been seen by man for over fifty years.

We pulled ourselves out of the water and lay shivering on the bank. When Stalking Wolf appeared at the edge of the stream, carrying with him two steaming hot cups of coffeelike liquid, we drank eagerly of the semi-bitter brew which warmed us deep to the very marrow. Chicory-root tea was one of our favorite cold-weather drinks from that time on. We would gather the roots in the fall, clean them well, then roast them in little stone ovens until they were brown and brittle. We stone-ground the root fibers until they were granulated, then used a small palmful of root grounds to a large cup of hot water. I love chicory tea with honey or mixed with mint teas.

I use the whitish underground part of new leaves and plants as a trailside nibble or a welcome addition to salads. I also love these little leafstalks lightly steamed, but still crisp, served like a vegetable. They are absolutely delicious. The new leaves can be cooked fresh in boiling water for five minutes. They make a good spinach substitute that is a welcome treat at any survival outing or dinner table. One of my favorite recipes is to cook the leafstalks and new leaves separately, mix them together, then add ground acorns and uncooked sliced mushrooms.

Medicinal Chicory leaves and flowers can be boiled and wrapped in a clean, cotton cloth. Still warm and wet, the cloth can be applied to swelling inflammations and boils. I also find it effective on mild infections. The strong tea made from boiling the roots, leaves, and flowers makes a good wash for skin irritations, such as poison ivy, bee stings, and even the discomforts of athlete's foot. I also use a milder tea as a mouthwash for cold sores and other abscesses. Its relief is instantaneous and long-lasting.

A good tonic drink can be made which is effective in increasing the appetite, aiding in digestion, and improving all-around health. Boil a small palmful of dried rootstock and a small palmful of dried leaves in one cup of water for five minutes. Take a half cup in the morning and a half cup before bedtime. Roots are best collected in the fall or early spring. For a strong tea used for medicinal purposes, the leaves should be of the older type, which are quite bitter. Milder teas can be made from the fresh, new leaves. A mild tea made from the new green leaves is good for settling an upset stomach. Use a good palmful of shredded green leaves to eight ounces of hot water and steep for twenty minutes.

Chickweed (*Stellaria spp.*)

Description   Most of the chickweeds are edible and medicinal, though the common chickweed is one of the best for both. It is a beautiful little plant of the moist soils, waste soils, and gardens. It may grow upright or in tangled, low-growing carpets. The uppermost part of a long stalk will sport a tiny white flower. Sometimes you will have to look very closely, because it is so dainty that it can easily be missed. Its leaves are paired and smooth, and it flowers for most of the season. The flower petals are deeply notched at the tip and longer than the sepals. Chickweed is found throughout the United States.

Personality   Not far from my boyhood home was a small grove of sourgum located in a lowland area. In a small clearing grew a lush patch of common chickweed, bathed continuously in the dampness of the forest. I would spend hours there on hot summer days, lying back on the mat of chickweed, which felt cool and refreshing against my bare skin. This little forest chapel was always damp and cool, giving me the overall feeling of being in the cellars of some old stone temple. It became a room separated from the rest of the world, with its own atmosphere and temperature so as to feel totally removed from the torrid heat just a few yards away. Those few yards could have been thousands of miles, for this place always relaxed the body and set the mind free to wander at will, uninhibited.

There, especially, Rick and I would role-play animals. Becoming an animal was important in the understanding of any particular animal so we would emulate them as closely as possible. Many times this role-playing would help us out of a tight tracking jam, when there were no visible tracks left to follow. Once when I was tracking, I lost the trail of a small rabbit at the foot of a large tangle of bullbrier. For hours I combed the ground looking for the slightest sign to indicate which way he had gone. Grandfather came by and suggested that we should think like the rabbit, which could give us a clue to where he might have gone. We tried thinking like that rabbit but to no avail. Upon his return trip he noticed that we had made no progress so he said that we shouldn't only think like the rabbit but actually become the rabbit. Look at the world as the rabbit does, feel what he feels, and rework with your body the trail scenario written before the brier patch.

Knowing that the rabbit had been frightened by a fox, we lay on our bellies and pretended that we were the rabbit wanting to escape. We got so involved in playing the rabbit that in our minds we actually became rabbits. Grandfather shouted and I dived down the smaller of the two trails instinctively. Laughing to the point of tears, he then asked me which way the rabbit would have gone. It was easily confirmed by the fresh tracks under my nose. As time progressed, we role-played animals frequently, walking as they did, moving through the brush as they did, and feeding as they did. This is why chickweed was so important to us, because we could forage on the succulent tops just like the deer, rabbits, and groundhogs did. We became the animals and the chickweed added that realistic essence of feeding.

Chickweed was one of the first plants for which I found the medicinal use by myself. It had been a particularly hot and humid day. I took refuge in the chickweed patch, where I could escape the heat and still get some writing done without sweating to death. The oppressive heat only increased with the day and did not show any signs of letting up in the evening, so I spent the entire day within the confines of the temple grove. I didn't even take a break to forage but just continuously fed on the cool succulent chickweed tops from early morning until just about the time I was to leave. I was so bloated by overeating that I could walk but halfway home. The bloated feeling was quickly relieved by the worse case of diarrhea I have had to this day.

By the end of summer, I had all but forgotten about my bout with the chickweed until Rick developed a bad case of constipation. We were hiking to one of Grandfather's camps to spend the weekend, and we wanted to get there before dark. The going was very slow because Rick, who had serious cramps and an upset stomach from the constipation, had to stop frequently to rest. When we stopped next to a chickweed patch, the memory of my diarrhea came rushing back. I figured that the chickweed might help Rick's problem, so I gathered a few handfuls. I realized that Rick would never be able to eat the chickweed with an upset stomach, so I would concentrate it in tea form. I added the chickweed to hot water, brewed a strong tea, and gave it to Rick to drink.

His cramping and upset stomach began to ease up shortly after the warm tea hit his stomach, and we continued with our hike. Unfortunately, as we got closer to camp, our pace was slowed again while Rick frequently had to relieve himself: His bowels had loosened up to the point of violent diarrhea. Grandfather was delighted over the way I had discovered the medicinal values of chickweed by myself. He taught us to use our own bodies as we ate any herbs, noting the feelings and changes so we could use the herbs later on as a possible medication. It was one of the ways the herbs could communicate with us and demand full attention.

Grandfather was not, however, pleased with the way I had overmedicated Rick. Rick's diarrhea continued over quite a few days, and we were forced to call off the rest of the campout. Grandfather lectured me on how haphazardly I had prescribed the medication. At best, I had only been interested in an overdose to clear up Rick's problem quickly, and had given no apparent thought to what the side effects of the medication would be. In this case, I had only made the problem worse; thus we still had to call off the campout. I did learn, however, that it is better to give a lower dose of medication and watch its effects. I could have always increased the dosage later on; and realistically, a gentler approach in this case would have saved Rick much aggravation.

Food   Chickweed can be eaten raw or added to salads. Only the new leaves and succulent tops of the plant should be eaten raw, however. Mouse-ear chickweed should always be cooked because of the hairiness of the leaves. One of the best ways to eat the chickweed is to steam it for five minutes and eat it like a potherb. Whole plants, except for the roots, can be used in the steaming process, which produces a unique and very palatable taste, a favorite with novice herbalists.

Chickweed has a refreshing taste whether it is eaten raw or cooked. Whenever I eat it, it reminds me of that chickweed patch of long ago and the quiet reprieve that it always gave me. In truth, I become so intimately involved with the plant people that it becomes difficult to separate the true physical taste from the emotional taste cultivated by experience. You will find that when you begin your quest to discover new plants the feelings, emotions, and experiences with the plant are every bit as important as the physical act of collection. This intimate knowledge of the plants expands the taste to include emotion and memory.

Medicinal   The most powerful use of chickweed is as a laxative. Take a palmful of fresh, chopped leaves, add to a cup of hot water, and let steep for one-half hour. Strain out the leaves through cheesecloth or a grass mat, and squeeze the remaining juices back into the hot liquid. Take one-half cup twice a day for constipation. If that dosage fails to loosen the bowels, then take one cup twice a day.

Mild tea made from the fresh leaves also has a certain decongestant property. It is mild, at best, but is effective in clearing up my sinus headaches. It will not dry out the nasal passages. Chopped leaves can be wrapped in a cloth, dipped in warm water, and applied directly to skin abrasions, boils, blisters, and bruises. The juices can also be added to tallow to form a good balm for chapped lips and weather-ravaged skin.

Chickweed, except for its laxative qualities, is a very mild medication. This tends to steer herbalists away from it as one of the healing herbs, but many times it is better to go to a mild medication rather then a strong one. Take, for instance, a sinus headache. A strong herb with antihistamine qualities will crack open and dry up your sinuses but will also dry out all your breathing apparatus. Dry nasal and trachea passages will not allow the cilia to work at sweeping out dust and germs, thus you leave yourself open to other, more serious complications. Better results can be obtained by using herbs with milder expectorant properties, opening the sinus without the dry-out factor. Many times, milder is better, especially when it comes to herbs.

Coltsfoot (*Tussilago farfara*)

Description   Coltsfoot is the flower of waste grounds. It is an elegant plant; the flowers are yellow and bristly in appearance, the rays having a layered effect. These grow on long, elegant stalks covered with reddish scales. In the spring, when the plant flowers, these stalks seem to grow directly from the ground, the basal leaves appearing after the flowers. The basal leaves are large and in a wavy heart shape, sometimes reaching eighteen inches in length. Coltsfoot grows throughout most of the Northeast, ranging as far south as Ohio, to New Jersey.

Personality   The name *coltsfoot* brings me back to medieval times when sorcerers and witches concocted strange brews and cast spells upon unsuspecting peasants. The plant's strange but simple appearance takes me to another time and place, of steamy swamps, thick forests, and mystical castles. When I was young, I looked at coltsfoot cautiously, thoroughly convinced that it belonged to the occult. I felt that it was one of those herbs that were taboo, off limits to us inexperienced naturalists. As I grew older, my fascination with the plant increased because I knew instinctively that it had power. However, I still felt that it was used for evil purposes. Every time I asked Grandfather about the plant, he just put me off. He said that I had to wait until I was older, when I had more herbal experience and could understand its power more. This only succeeded in arousing only more curiosity, and I held the plant in even more mystical awe.

All my suspicions about coltsfoot were confirmed one day while I was collecting cattail roots from our local swamp. I spied a movement in an open forest that bordered the outer area of the swamp. Feeling that it might be a deer foraging, I stalked closer to get a better look. To my shock, an old woman was collecting plants, softly singing to herself in a high shrill voice, some strange song that bordered on a chant. Chills ran up my spine when I realized that it was the old woman who lived on the other side of the swamp. This same woman was said to hold seances, perform strange healings, and otherwise be possessed with the devil. Rick and I always steered clear of her home because we knew that she was a witch, probably involved in some black magic that utilized little boys as sacrifices.

I could not get close enough to see exactly what kind of plant she was collecting so I waited, hoping that she would soon leave. I was well concealed in the brush and quite confident of the fact that she could not see me. My illusion was broken when she picked up her basket and bags, began to walk down the trail, then stopped and waved back at me. Her old face and toothless grin sent chills through my body, and I ran, crashing through brush until I collapsed, exhausted. There was no way she could have seen me in the brush for I had been very quiet and was accomplished at camouflage to the point where most animals would pass me by. The old woman's knowing where I was hidden was proof positive that she possessed some extrasensory ability, definitely witchcraft.

I found Rick at his house and breathlessly told him the story. My greatest fear was that since she knew I was there and had seen some of her secrets, she would cast a voodoo spell on me, and I would surely perish. A few days passed, and I was delighted that I had not come down with some strange sickness and my luck was still good. My curiosity got the better of me when Rick asked me what kind of plant she had been collecting and I didn't know. We went back to the forest and began to track the old woman to the place where she had been collecting. Our suspicions were confirmed when we found that she had been collecting coltsfoot. Truly, we thought, this plant was used for all the evil purposes we had imagined.

Weeks passed, and thoughts of the witch had been long lost in the hollows of my mind. Then one day, Grandfather asked us to accompany him on a trip to the house of another herbal healer. He had to pick up some plants that he needed for his medicine bundle, and he wanted us to meet someone very special. I broke into a cold sweat and my heart began to pound as we approached the house of the witch. I began badgering Grandfather not to go any farther, describing the events of the plant-collecting and stating that everyone thought she was a witch. I explained that no one with normal powers could have seen me in the woods and no one I knew of, except for Rick and me, was ever interested in herbs, especially the dreaded coltsfoot.

Reluctantly I approached the house, full of apprehension but overwhelmed with curiosity and excitement. The old witch appeared at the door and gave Grandfather a warm smile. Grandfather introduced Rick and me, describing us as his apprentices and explaining our interest in plants and the natural world. She smiled, looked at me, and said, "We meet again." She went on to say that maybe I shouldn't be so afraid of rumors and others' opinions of her. I was delighted to find that she was not a witch at all, but an experienced herbalist and midwife, quite well-known throughout these parts.

Grandfather had arranged our meeting not only to introduce us to her, but also for us to begin to learn with her. Instinctively, from that day on, we began to call her Grandmother.

With the formalities, and my fears, done away with, I began to ask questions. Still with reservation, I asked about the spooky colts-foot and described in detail my greatest thoughts and fears about the plant. Grandmother only laughed and said that coltsfoot was no more dangerous than she was. I had allowed myself to bend to superstition, outward appearances, and what other people had said. Thus I was prejudiced and could not allow myself to learn of the plant because of unfounded fears. She also said that I should learn to make judg-ments for myself about plants as well as people. I should never listen to hearsay because it would only stand in the way of the possibilities of deeper friendships. Lesson learned, we began to discover the beauty and powers of coltsfoot, which surpassed our wildest imagination.

Our first encounter with the edible properties of coltsfoot came in the form of tea. During our get-acquainted talk, Grandmother served us a delicious tea. Its flavor was remarkable, soothing, and very pow-erful. It had qualities that reached beyond mere mortal description and could only fully be expressed with the emotions. After a few cups, Grandmother asked us how we liked the coltsfoot. Almost sub-consciously, I began to grow sick to my stomach as all my fears of the plant welled up once again. Visibly, I must have turned pale because she commented that I was allowing past superstitions to interfere with my judgment. Instantly, I began to feel better, squelch-ing any thought or preconceived ideas and allowing the beautiful essence of the plant to return.

Grandmother was with us many years, and we visited her quite often. We became her grandchildren, and her knowledge flowed to us openly and without restriction. We even accompanied her when we were older to a few natural childbirths and observed the beautiful bedside manner for which she was known. Her love and friendship to all her patients was always flowing. She spread hope and peace wherever she went, the physical embodiment of true brotherhood and love. She was famous with the children, for she always listened to their stories and, most of all, brought her delicious candy, made from coltsfoot.

Food   One of my first survival experiences with coltsfoot was a delight. We had been camping for quite some time, our aim being to seek out the spiritual levels instead of the survival levels. We had, at best, a meager shelter and just enough foraged food. We were on a controlled fast from all things comfortable. After seven days of this ascetic existence, we began to build our camp, the height of our devotions now over. Both Rick and I were quite hungry and in need of a good meal. The entire week had been spent on a bland diet, and now we wanted something more substantial. After camp was built up and put in order, we went out to hunt.

Within a few minutes, Rich bagged himself a nice fat cottontail. Back at camp we cooked it up by roasting it in a stone oven. We began to feast on the rabbit when Rick said that he would love to have some salt. Salt is one of the first things that people miss on a survival outing, and both of us wished that we had some. It would break the monotony of our rather bland diet. Grandfather simply stated that there was enough salt contained in our diet and that we really needed no more. What we were craving was the taste of the salt on the meat.

The rabbit was set by the fire, and we followed Grandfather on a short walk to the edge of our camp. He promised that we would be delighted to learn something new about an old plant friend, something that would enhance our meal. A short distance from camp, he found some coltsfoot and gathered a handful of the larger leaves. We took these back to camp and laid them close to the fire to dry quickly. He then put them onto a clean piece of bark and slowly burned them until they turned into a pile of black ash. He sprinkled the ash onto our rabbit and told us to eat. To our delight, the ash tasted very similar to salt, only not as biting. We were thrilled as we sat and ate, breaking the back of a bland diet, and talking about all the ways we could use the saltlike coltsfoot in our recipes.

The dried leaves of coltsfoot can be used to make a fine tea. Candy can be made by adding one cup of chopped fresh leaves to one cup of water, then simmering for one-half hour. Strain the leaves through a cheesecloth or woven grass screen, and save the extract. Add two cups of sugar to every cup of extract. Boil the mixture until thick and rich. Slowly drop the hot syrup in small clumps into cold water. Hard balls of candy will form. I prefer brown sugar for this recipe, though I do not recommend the consumption of large amounts of any sugar. If the boiling time of the candy recipe is cut short, the resulting syrup can be used for a glaze on baked meat dishes or for a topping on ice cream. It is also good in tea or coffee and, of course, on pancakes.

Medicinal To make a good astringent or skin wash, bring two cups of water to a boil. Add two cups of mature green leaves, and remove from the heat. Let steep for one hour, strain, and wipe directly on bee stings, poison ivy rash, mild cuts and abrasions, and other skin maladies. For stronger astringent effects on unbroken skin, use one cup of chopped green leaves and one cup of chopped root to a cup and a half of water. Bring to a boil and let steep for two hours.

Coltsfoot also makes a good cough remedy, which has an expectorant property. It can be used for hoarseness, for soothing a sore throat, and for alleviating any other type of cough. A cough tea can be made by adding fresh coltsfoot flowers and chopped mature green leaves to hot water and steeping for thirty minutes. Strain, then drink like a tea. Use a palmful of the herb to one cup of water as the usual tea dose, taken twice a day. To make a cough syrup, steep three cups of freshly-chopped leaves in two cups of hot water for two hours. Do not boil. Strain out the leaves, add two cups of brown sugar to one cup of extract, and simmer to a syruplike consistency. This is best taken warm four times a day. Further boiling until it turns into a thick, rich, syrup produces a cough drop when cooled.

One of the last medicinal uses I learned for coltsfoot was in the later years of my apprenticeship with Grandfather. We had a small overnight camp set up and were preparing for a ceremony that was to take place at sunrise. The late fall air was cold and damp, the kind of cold that penetrated the clothing and body right to the marrow. I was on the upswing of a bad chest cold and could not stop coughing. The tightness in my chest felt as if all my bronchial tubes were clogged, and the coughing hurt deep inside. I had used the regular cough medicines, but to no avail, and I felt destined to cough right through the sunrise ceremony.

As we sat at the fire that night, the conversation was continually broken by my hacking. At times it felt as if I could hardly get my breath. Grandfather rummaged around in his bag and finally brought out a buckskin pouch filled with what I thought was tobacco. He methodically packed his personal pipe, then lit it. He passed the pipe to me, instructing me to take the smoke deep into my lungs. I smoked for a while then passed the pipe back to Grandfather, never realizing that I had just taken a medication. We talked well into the night when I suddenly realized that I had hardly coughed and that the congestion in my lungs had broken up. Realizing that the cough had stopped after I smoked the pipe, I asked Grandfather what it was. He answered, "Coltsfoot leaves."

Comfrey (*Symphytum officinale*)

Description   Comfrey, a lover of the waste places, is found along roadsides, ditches, and in old fields. It is a hairy plant, coarse in appearance with alternate spear-shaped leaves that taper to a winged stem. The flowers come in soft purple, yellow, pink, or white, are five-lobed and bell-shaped. The flowers appear as a curling cluster on a curved stem. Preceding the cluster is a pair of winglike leaves. Throughout the summer it flowers. It grows from Ontario and the northeastern United States, ranging as far south as Georgia.

Personality   My first encounter with comfrey was on an emergency level. I had just returned from a week-long summer campout that my parents had no idea I was on. I was supposed to be spending the week at Rick's house and he at mine, as we normally did to buy ourselves longer periods of time in the woods. The tension this created was ridiculous, but we would go on with the campout anyway, hoping that neither set of our parents would get in touch with the other. We always meticulously prepared ourselves for the return trip by bringing clean clothes with us. That way we did not look like we had been in the woods at all. Unfortunately, I was at the age where I had to shave at least every other day, and as a result of shaving, I met the comfrey plant.

We were all cleaned up and on our way home when I decided to shave. I figured that if I were clean shaven, my parents would have not even the slightest clue that I had been anywhere other than Rick's. I remember hearing about the old mountain men shaving with their knives, so I thought that this would be a golden opportunity to try it myself. I didn't have a razor anyway, so it even gave me more of an excuse. I sharpened my knife to a keen edge, buffed up some meadowsweet soap, and began to shave at the stream. I did rather well and was virtually done until I decided to trim my sideburns. That was when I slipped slightly and gave myself a rather long and bloody razor cut.

It just would not stop bleeding, no matter how much pressure we put against the wound. It was located in a place where, whenever I opened my mouth, it would separate. I was forced to walk home with a wad of old cloth pressed against my face. Grandmother was in her garden when she saw us walk by. She noticed the rag on the side of my head and asked if I had a toothache. We explained the whole bloody story and how I feared that I would get in trouble at home for doing such a stupid thing. I was sure that my folks would find out that I had been out in the woods; and if my mother ever saw the blood, I would be confined to a life of mediocrity until I turned twenty-one. Any damage to her son's body was always blamed on the woods, and I didn't want to take any chances.

Grandmother took me into her house, washed the wound and lovingly inspected it to see that it wasn't too deep. She removed a small glass jar from the shelf and set it on the table. Carefully she removed a tiny bit of powder from it and inspected it closely to see that it looked clean. Holding the powder in a soft cotton cloth, she began to dab it onto my wound, and magically stopped the bleeding. There was no pain from the powder. Within minutes, she had cleaned me up to a point where the cut looked like any other of the small scrapes we frequently got in the woods. Her only request for healing me was that we gather her more comfrey the next time we were in her area.

It was unfortunate that the cut on my face now looked as if it were a small scrape from a stick. As soon as my dad saw the scrape, we were suspected of escaping to the woods, and a call of confirmation to Rick's parents got us grounded for a week. We were chomping at the bit to get out in the woods to collect that comfrey and learn all about it from Grandmother. Every time we passed each other in school that week, we would discuss the plant and all the possibilities it had. In our free time, we would go into the library and read anything we could get our hands on that might give us a clue to the power of comfrey.

Comfrey is one of those plants whose tremendous power you instinctively know. Even the way it looks suggests a plant that must have healed people for centuries. If you let your imagination run wild, the flowers look like the head of a dragon bent to the ground; and the leaves near the flowers look like wings. To see a whole patch of these healthy plant people is to look into a flock of white, yellow, pink, purple, and blue dragons. Even the color variations in the flowers created a mystery that kept us baffled with the whys of it all for weeks. To us, comfrey begged to be discovered, understood, and known intimately as a powerful brother.

Food There is a place down by the river, a damp open forest that we call the comfrey dragon grove. It was there that we first spied Grandfather collecting the young greens of some new plant that we did not know. I can still close my eyes and see him in the mist, drifting about like some shadowy cloud, singing and talking to the plants. He had a grand way of teaching and riveting our attention to exactly what he wanted. He never forced us into anything but had us continually begging for knowledge. He never asked us to learn anything specific, but worked out things so that the piece of information he wanted to teach was all we wanted in life. His was a teaching that enticed us to learn. The little comfrey plants were no exception.

The collecting of the comfrey plants followed his way of teaching. He lured us to the plants with the mystery of what he was collecting. The mist and the songs added to the overall ambience and raised our curiosity. I wished more of my teachers at school would make me want to learn and make learning fun. Everyone likes to learn provided that the lesson is an adventure and the acquired knowledge is worth having. Stimulation and excitement about a subject make learning easier and the retaining of information longer. That is one of the key factors in getting to know about our plant brothers. It isn't something you just go out and do. There is too much information to learn, eventually lose, and possibly abuse. Learning about plants must be a need and a labor of love.

From the moment we saw Grandfather collecting the little plants in the lowlands, we needed to know all about them. He baited us with the things the plants could do and how they tasted. The more he talked, the more we wanted to learn. Our excitement built, not with his words but through his actions. His excitement, which took over his whole person, became contagious. Eagerly, we watched every step of the preparation, savoring each measure with our senses so that it was assimilated into the very fiber of our understanding. Tasting the plant was a ritual that we did with all the senses so that we knew the essence and spirit of the plant on all levels.

I learned the edible properties of the comfrey long before Grandmother introduced me to the medicinal ones. The newest leaves of early spring can be cooked like spinach. All the leaves are hairy but this hairyness disappears in cooking. Later on in the season, the older leaves can be eaten, provided they are cooked in several changes of water. The bitterness is cooked out in this process. As time goes by, you will find that only two changes of water are necessary, since you will develop a taste for wild things. I prefer a slightly bitter taste to some of my greens, and comfrey is one of my favorites. When we taste the first comfrey of the season, we know that spring is here to stay. The dried leaves also make a delicious tea. The young leaves make an excellent tea, but I prefer the stronger teas made from the older leaves.

Medicinal The comfrey root is where most of its medicinal values are stored. I collect the root in the early spring or late fall, as the plant begins to die off. The rootstock collected in summer has a milder medicinal value and can be used when milder remedies are indicated. Collect the root and allow it to partially dry in the warm afternoon sun. Scrape away the dark outer layer and slice the inner core into long flat strips. Allow the rootstocks to dry slowly in a cool dry place until they can be ground easily. Grind the rootstock with a mortar and pestle and store in a glass, earthenware, or clay container.

The powder of the rootstock can be applied directly to wounds that refuse to stop bleeding. It has a marvelous hemostatic property and, most of the time, helps the cut to heal with no scarring. Do not use it on large, gaping wounds, as it would take too much powder to cut off the bleeding and infection could occur. Make sure the powder is kept very clean because impure powder will cause infection.

For a strong medication, simmer a small palmful of powdered root in a cup of water for two to four minutes and let steep for thirty minutes. This can be taken two to three times a day for digestive problems, diarrhea, ulcers, and as a cough medication. This tea can also be used as a mouthwash for soothing sore throats, hoarseness, bleeding gums, and abscesses. It can also be used as a skin wash because it has great astringent properties and promotes healing of wounds. Crushed and simmered roots can be used as a poultice for bruises, boils, bee stings, and poison ivy. It also has a soothing effect on arthritis and rheumatism in some people. I also have found good results with the poultice on sprains and pulled tendons.

A milder tea can be made by soaking a good palmful of crushed or powdered root in one cup of cold water for six hours. Though some of the properties of the tea are diminished, its cough-suppressant and throat-soothing abilities vastly increase. This tea should be drunk warm, one cup twice a day. I found that this tea works well on persistent coughs that other cough medications will not touch. A good cough tonic is made by taking one-half cup of the root tea with one-half cup of the leaf tea, three times a day. Grandfather used to keep this tea mixture in powdered form in a buckskin bag. His tea mix was made with one-half rootstock powder and one-half broken, dried leaves. The tea was made by soaking leaves in hot water for one-half hour, straining and then taken twice a day. Sometimes dried and crushed rose hips were added to the bag for a good all-around cold remedy, available throughout the winter months.

Dandelion (*Taraxacum officinale*)

Description The word *dandelion* is derived from a French term meaning "tooth of a lion," referring to the plant's sharp lobes that appear as teeth on the leaves. The stems of dandelion are hollow and milky when broken. The seed balls are round, white, and downy. The flowerhead, solitary, is a beautiful yellow cluster of petals. It is found in disturbed soils around roadsides and lawns, especially favoring low grassy areas. It flowers from early spring to mid-fall, sometimes into the warmer days of winter. Dandelion grows throughout the United States.

Personality Fields of dandelion are like huge cloud rafts floating on a sea of green. Lying back on this flowery bed can become intoxicating, the mind swooning with the fragrance. Dandelions conjure up images of spring, their fresh scents so alluring, drawing one to run barefoot across their faces until the feet are green and yellow striped. It is also the lone flower of sunny winter places, defiantly blooming next to patches of mid-winter snow, always reminding us, even at the coldest times, that there is hope for spring. The close view of the flower itself creates an image of a fiery yellow explosion that originates from a common green heart. The myriad petals forming the rich golden-yellow crown seem to fire off in every direction, yet in perfect harmony, creating a balance of unity and common understanding.

Because of its zest for life, especially on grass, the dandelion has become a bane to the manicured lawn. For some reason, mankind hates any lawn that is speckled with yellow. After all, lawns are meant to be totally green and uniform, like some manufactured carpet. Grandfather was not the first to introduce us to the dandelion. An elderly gentleman who had immigrated to this country from Italy when he was a young man made this introduction. He lived a few towns over from where we camped, so we had to pass his home on our way to the camp. One spring day we watched him weeding his lawn, pulling out dandelions and placing them into a large basket. We could almost feel the plants scream as they were pulled out of the flow of life. At least he was leaving the root for future generations.

We felt as if we were the warriors of the Earth, put there for her protection. We nervously set about telling this old man how we felt about the plants being needlessly killed. I felt that if we could just convince one person, then possibly, more would come around to our way of thinking. We had to start somewhere, and the old man with the funny accent seemed harmless enough. Confronting him, we said that we could not understand how anyone could feel that the dandelion was ugly or that it made a lawn look bad. After all, there was no such thing as a weed. He only smiled at us and waved us onto his porch where we thought we would get another lecture on the virtues of killing weeds for the betterment of the Earth.

Instead he sat us down and smiled at us with a big toothy grin. He asked if we were thirsty and if we would like some fine wine. Being rebels and knowing that alcohol was off-limits to us, we jumped at the chance to taste some. Anything off-limits was automatically enticing and very desirous. He gave us two small glasses of a pale, golden wine poured from an unlabeled bottle. The taste fascinated us, for it went beyond the mere senses, tasting as light and refreshing as a mild spring day. We talked for hours but never had another glass of the wine until we finally set aside our pride and asked for more. After we had savored the wine and were about to leave, we asked what kind of wine it was. The old man smiled and simply said, "Dandelion."

We were shocked. Losing all thought of protocol, we bombarded him with questions, just as we would have done with Grandfather. We begged him to show us how to make the wine, what part of the plant was used, and how it was harvested. The old man must have been starved for this type of attention, and we ended up staying the whole day and well into the night. We worked in the basement of his home, helping him to prepare the flowers and taking part in the winemaking. Ironically, we sat down to dinner at his table that night only to drink more wine, eat dandelion greens and dandelion flowers made into fritters. We finished off the meal with a tea made from the roots of the plant which he called dandelion coffee.

We were amazed. Here was a man who we had passed for months and a flower that we had known for years, both coming together to teach us. Every week on the way to the camp area, we would stop and learn from this old man we lovingly called Gramps. He seemed to have a wealth of knowledge, especially about the Old World plants that had taken root in this country. His wisdom seemed limitless, and we estimated that he could probably find a thousand uses for any plant. Unfortunately, in the fall of that same year, he passed away to the other side. All the knowledge he had now seemed hopelessly lost. We grew angry at ourselves for not spending more time with him.

As we passed his house later that fall, a younger man was in the front yard picking the last of the blooming dandelions. A FOR SALE sign sat squarely at the corner of the house. The man looked much like a younger version of Gramps. We were excited beyond words; could this be Gramps's son, picking the dandelions for another batch of that springlike wine? We ran to the house and began asking the man questions, finding, to our delight, that he was in fact the oldest son of Gramps. Our hearts seemed to be pulled from our chest when we found that he was weeding the lawn instead of making wine. After all, the house had to be sold, and a yellow-spangled lawn was undesirable.

Before we left, realizing that we were the two boys that his father had written to him about, he handed us an old book. It was Gramp's journal of herbs and remedies, written over the past few decades. Inscribed in the front were our names, thanking us for listening to this strange old man and how it made his heart soar. I cried, realizing how many old, knowledgeable people are out there locked away in nursing homes and forgotten, needing so desperately to talk to anyone who would listen. I vowed that I would always seek out the old ones and listen to their wisdom. From that day forward, one of my greatest delights has been to visit the old and forgotten whenever I can.

We found out later that Gramps was ninety-seven years old, not sixty-two as everyone thought. In his journal he had written that he attributed his long life to four things: his unfailing belief and devotion to the Creator, dandelion wine, dandelion tonic, and listening to everyone as a teacher. From that day on, we always referred to Gramps as Grandpa Dandelion. I never pass a dandelion today that I don't think of him, on his hands and knees on the lawn, his fine dandelion wine, and his loving but lonely eyes.

Food   Every fall, Grandfather, Rick, and I would set about the long and deliberate ritual of making our dandelion coffee stock for the coming winter. We would wander about old lawns and waste areas looking for just the right plants with the best roots. Small roots were not tasty enough, and large roots made a slightly bitter brew. What we were after was the medium-sized but fat roots that would produce the best taste. We took great care in our collecting, making sure to scatter any of the seedheads that were in bloom, and saving all the edible parts. We carefully placed the roots in a large basket and covered them with damp grasses.

Back at camp, we would then start the coffee-making procedure. After washing the roots carefully and removing all blemishes and old cuts, we would let them dry slightly for six hours in the mild fall sun.

While they were drying, we would collect some local sandstone and build small square ovens facing a fire-pit area. We would then build a fire, building up a thick bed of coals, and place the dandelion roots into the oven. We would allow them to cook slowly overnight until they were a rich dark brown and quite brittle.

The next day we would lay the roots out in the warm fall sun again as we began to grind the roots with a stone mortar and pestle. The grinds would be placed on a traylike basket and kept in the full sun, just to make sure that no moisture remained in the grinds. By mid-afternoon, before the day grew damp, we would place the grinds in buckskin bags or in pottery bowls with tight lids. These would be sealed with beeswax and placed in a cool and dry place inside our shelters for winter use. Sometimes we would also make a blend of coffee using half chicory-root grinds and half dandelion-root grinds. Other unique coffeelike brews can be made by adding one-third dried mint leaves, or one-third green pine needles, or one-third dried yarrow leaves.

The brewing process was almost as intricate a procedure as making dandelion wine. We would burn out the inside of a log with coals, then carve it into the shape of a funnel, or make a pottery bowl with tiny holes punched in the bottom as our dandelion grind holder. Our filter was made out of a fine mesh weave of grass or the inner bark of cedar, which was placed inside the holder. The grinds were then placed inside the holder, a good-sized palmful to every cup of water. We would then boil some water and pour it slowly over the grinds, allowing it to drain into the cup. If a stronger brew was desired, the first brew was recycled for a second or third time, depending on how strong we wanted our finished product. Dandelion coffee became one of our winter staples and would go with us wherever we went.

The tender, young leaves, still pale green in color, can be added raw to salads or cooked for five minutes in boiling water and eaten like a pot herb. The tender whitish stalks of these leaves make an excellent trailside nibble, or can be cooked the same way the young leaves are prepared. If the herb tastes too bitter, pour off the first boiling and simmer again for five minutes. This should get rid of the bitter taste. The flowerheads, before they erupt into bloom, can be boiled from five to ten minutes in two changes of water and eaten like brussels sprouts. Covered with melted cheese, they make a good vegetable for dinner. The flowers are excellent dipped in grass seed or acorn batter, then deep fried in tallow and eaten like a fritter.

Dandelion is a good friend to the survivalist and a beautiful addition to the bouquet of wildflowers covering the Earth. It is not a common weed, as most lawn owners will suggest, but a welcome addition to the beauty of the land, our health, and our tables. There is no such thing as a weed, just people's weedy misconception of life creatures and how they fit into society's world.

Medicinal The dandelion is one of the great all-around medicinals for maintaining good health when used as a tonic. A tonic is made by steeping a small palmful of leaves in one cup of hot water. Take one-half cup in the morning and one-half cup in the evening. Milder tonics can be made from the dried young leaves. A stronger tonic can be made from the young, green leaves. Stronger tonics also have stimulant and diuretic properties. The mild teas aid in digestion and sometimes relieve stomach cramps. Dandelion leaves are also very high in vitamin A. When added to salads, they make a great health food.

Elderberry (*Sambucus canadensis*)

Description   The elderberry is a lover of rich damp soils, especially streambanks, ditches, and wet thickets. Its beautiful white flower clusters appear in early summer. Its tiny purple fruits appear in early fall. Leaves are divided into five- to eleven-toothed leaflets; the twigs are soft and thick, with a dense white pith. It is a full, erect shrub, and from the distance, the flower clusters appear as a haze over the bushes. The elderberry is found in much of the northeastern United States and into Canada. Its range also extends south into Georgia and Louisiana.

Personality   We had been working on our personal pipes for days. For more than a week, we had wandered about the scrub oak groves, looking for a suitable piece of wood that would make a good bowl. We had gathered some fire-killed oak that was growing along an old roadway, and were quite pleased with the shape and personalities of our would-be pipe bowls. Every evening, we carved and sanded our pipes, finally staining them a deep walnut color, using some walnut husks that we had collected up north. With the bowls now done, we set about making the stems. Wandering in groves of cedar, we selected some suitable pipe staves and began to hollow them out.

We first tried burning out the stems using tiny coals, then abrading away the char with a small pump drill. We burned through quite a few before we eventually gave up. We split the remaining pipestems and scraped out a trough in the centers, then bound those together with pitch glue and rawhide. The results were crude but serviceable. Eventually, the stems grew too hot, melting the pitch, and filling our mouths with the burning resins of the melting glue. We gave up and only smoked the pipes when we were brave enough to withstand the vapors. Needless to say, we smoked rarely.

Grandfather observed our whole procedure with his usual amused attitude. After we came to him with our complaints, he told us of a few plants that had hollow cores and would make excellent pipe stems. One such plant was elderberry, which had been planted in an old farm field not far from where we were camping. Though the plant stem would make a good pipe stem, it wasn't a strong stem and would have to be replaced every few months. But we were delighted over the prospects of finding an almost ready-made stem, so we set out to find the elderberry bush.

We collected a few old dead stems, so as not to hinder the

growing plant. We found that the inside was easily removed by pushing a sharp oak stick down through the pith. Furthermore, we carved and decorated the stem quite easily. My first stem lasted almost a year (until I got careless and inadvertently sat on the pipe). We found many other uses for the stems, our favorite being a straw to suck up water from a drinking hole. Candles could also be made by soaking the hollow stems in tallow and lighting one end. These burned slowly and with more than adequate light. A hand-drill apparatus for making fires and blowguns could also be made from the stems. All in all, it was a great little survival plant.

The elderberry stems were eventually replaced by the stronger sumac stems in most cases, but these were more difficult to hollow out. Elderberry was still the stem of choice in a survival situation where speed was necessary. Though elderberry was first known to us as a utilitarian plant, it wasn't long before we learned more about this plant brother. It was during one of the times we were collecting the stems for blowguns that I first was introduced to another use of the plant. This started a fascination with the elderberry bush that has not left me to this day.

We had hiked a long way from camp in the hot sun, taking quite a few hours to reach the elderberry patch. We wanted to collect some tubing for blowguns and a few stems for hand drills. By the time we arrived at the area, I had a pounding headache that was making me sick to my stomach. Grandfather asked me to lie down in the bush itself while he prepared a medication. In the confines of the bush, the atmosphere was very cooling. Because of the bush's thick canopy, very little vegetation grew beneath, and the place seemed like a small, quiet, and cool room. It was a soothing place where the tranquillity of the room and the reprieve from the hot sun made my head feel much better.

As I lay on my back, I watched Grandfather gather a handful of the flowers, removing the petals carefully from the green. He placed the flowers in a cup of hot water and allowed them to steep for about a half hour. He gave me the cup to drink slowly as I relaxed inside the natural shelter. Almost immediately, my upset stomach began to clear up and soon after, the headache lost its power over me. As I relaxed in the bush, allowing the medication to work, I couldn't help but feel the connection of the soothing confines of the bush to the soothing medication it produced. Within a half hour, all the symptoms of the headache, the upset stomach, and the fatigue that went along with it had disappeared. I felt better than ever, and I even had more energy than I had in a long time.

Lying in the quiet room of the bush was a way of communication. I should have known, or at least felt, that the plant was trying to communicate with me. If I had stopped long enough to feel what the plant was telling me, I could have understood the parallel between the feeling and the potential medication. It is in this subtle way that most plants try to communicate with us, providing that we can relax enough to listen. The laying aside of the logical mind and the opening of the spiritual mind set in action the inner mechanism of communication, so necessary to understanding the subtle voices of nature.

Food The stems, roots, leaves, and unripe berries of the elderberry plant can cause vomiting, diarrhea, and general stomach upset. In some people they can cause even more discomfort or serious maladies. However, there are parts of the elderberry bush that are very edible. The ripe fruit makes an excellent cold drink. Boil the berries for fifteen minutes in water, mash them, then boil again. Strain the juice through cheesecloth or grass filters, chill and serve as a cold drink. Some people do not like the smell or taste of the juice so it is best to mix fifty-fifty with other sweeter juices until the taste can be acquired. Jelly can be made from the berry juices, but commercial pectin or gelatin from greenbrier root should be added to promote jelling.

The flower clusters can be dipped in batter and deep fried to make delicious fritters. The berries are usually rank smelling and unpleasant tasting, but this can be easily remedied. Drying the berries on trays in the warm sun will remove the poor taste and smell. These dried berries can then be reconstituted in boiling water and used in ash cakes, pancakes, and as fillings for the famous elderberry pies. These dried berries are easily stored for winter use. We would make pemmican out of one-third tallow, one-third jerky, and one-third reconstituted elderberries. Elderberries are rich in vitamins C and A.

Caution: *I do not recommend elderberries to people with known food allergies.*

Medicinal My first medicinal experience with elderberry was in the form of a headache remedy that worked well. Not long after, I watched Grandfather treat a local farmer with the same plant but for entirely different ailments. Grandfather made a strong flower tea to induce sweating and clear up a headache due to a bad cold the farmer had had for quite a few days. The cold symptoms had all but disappeared by the next day. Another time, I saw Grandfather treat a bad burn by mixing berry syrup and tallow into an ointment and applying it directly to a burn. The burn healed without any visible scarring, and quite quickly at that. To make the syrup, he crushed then boiled down a cup of berries, then strained and boiled again until a rich syrup was produced. To this, he added tallow until it reached a puddinglike consistency. The remedy was very soothing to all burns, including sunburn, and I have used it with great results on chafing.

The dried berries can be added to water and boiled into a rich tea. Take one-half cup of dried berries to two cups of water and simmer for ten minutes. To alleviate diarrhea, take the tea cold, one-half cup twice a day. A tea made from one cup of dried leaves simmered in two cups of water for ten minutes produces a good skin wash for any skin malady. It is especially effective on bee stings, sunburn, acne, and scrapes. I find that if a paste is made by mixing tallow with the tea, it produces a good drawing salve for boils and splinters.

Evening Primrose (*Oenothera biennis*)

Description   The evening primrose is a beautiful plant that has a long reddish stem and is sometimes branched. It produces a low rosette of leaves the first year and a flowerstalk the second. The plant is very leafy, rough, and hairy. The beautiful yellow flowers are four petaled and have a distinctive X-shaped stigma. They are at the end of a slender tube, rising from the swollen ovaries. They bloom from June to October. These plants are lovers of roadsides, dry soil, and waste ground. They grow in much of the eastern and central United States and may be found as far west as North Dakota and Idaho.

Personality   It was Grandpa Dandelion who first introduced us to evening primrose. We were out working on his garden when we spied a small patch of these plants growing by the edge of a dirt road. He was delighted at his discovery, for they were a source of food in the early spring and middle fall. He told us that he had planted the seeds a few years before and had forgotten about them. Now they were in their second year, sporting an elegant reddish flowerstalk that bore quite a few buds. He explained that they would bloom in the evening, then wilt by the next day, thus explaining their name. We were excited at the prospect, and for a few days, the plants became the center of our attention.

Every evening, for the better part of the week, we would sit by the primrose patch watching the swollen flower buds. We were sure that at any time the flowers would explode into bloom, and we wanted to be there to enjoy them. We were like guests at an opening night performance, the stars being the primrose flowers. Rick had borrowed his father's Brownie camera to take a few pictures, and I had my notebook ready to record the event in a crude form of poetry. We speculated what it must be like for a father awaiting the birth of his baby, comparing our wait to his. As the days passed by, our interest did not diminish but grew to an exciting anticipation like we had never felt before.

One morning while on our way to camp, I noticed a wilting yellow bloom in the primrose patch. We had missed the first bloom which must have come the night before after we left. We knew then that the others would be blooming that evening, so we went back to our homes to get our camping equipment. We were determined to camp there all night if necessary, so no other budding flower would escape us. We set up camp as if we were a scientific expedition to a foreign land. Our camera was set on a makeshift tripod, and I was standing by with my notebook. Spread before us was an assortment of tweezers, magnifying glasses, and field guides, all ready for the blessed event.

About two hours before sunset the flowers began to open. At first, only one moved and we thought that that was all there would be, but then another, and another, until a dozen began to move. Our eyes played tricks on us; we were hypnotized by the slow movement. We began to see things that did not exist, movements where there were none. There were far too many to see all at once; but we gave it a good try, finding that the more we moved our eyes from flower to flower and the less we tried to see the movement, the more movement we saw. The sequence of events was fascinating. At first, the bloom would move slightly, followed by the initial burst, then finally the slow movement of petals to the fully open position. When this was complete, the inner parts of the plant would arrange themselves to create the perfect blossom.

For us, just seeing the flowers open and then wilt the following morning was enough to give the plant tremendous spiritual value. Grandpa Dandelion was impressed at our dedication and discipline, so he went on to teach us things about this beautiful plant. The knowledge increased the plant's intrigue tremendously, and we fell in love with its taste. The first taste we had was right there the night the flowers opened. Grandpa Dandelion brought out a fresh garden salad garnished with his own homemade wild edible dressing. He dished out the salad then took a young and tender leaf from the tip of one of our plants. He peeled back the outer shell by scraping it with his knife, broke it up and added it to the salad. It gave a rich peppery taste to the salad and it was delicious. We used these peppery leaves in much of our cooking, like a spice.

Food   Grandfather also taught us a lot about primrose. The cooked roots were one of his favorite dishes, and he would go far out of his way to collect them. A few months after our first experience with the blooming primroses, Grandfather introduced us to more uses. We were on our way to the bulrush swamp when he took a side trip that led us to a patch of primrose a mile from the road. He searched through the patch and began digging up the roots of the plants that were in their first-year growth. The roots were carrotlike and pale pink, with a rich scent all their own.

We carried the roots to the camp area, then set up the camp while Grandfather scraped the outer cover off the roots. He cut the roots into round slices and boiled them for about half an hour, changing the water three times. They were absolutely delicious with a rich, pungent odor and a unique taste. Grandfather ate the primrose root sprinkled with coltsfoot salt and garnished with its own peppery leaves. At home, I loved to smother them in butter and soon enjoyed them more than potatoes or carrots. I tried mashing them though with little success, for they have a different consistency than potatoes, but they are still very good.

During the summer, the roots become quite peppery, but in the fall and spring, they are less so. I also add a small amount of fresh root to my salads as a spice. I boil the new green leaves for one-half hour in two changes of water. I like their powerful taste, but some people feel that they are too strong. Taste varies from person to person, and usually, the more experience you have with wild edibles, the more you prefer the stronger tastes. When we were learning, Grandfather had us at least sample everything, even though we may not have liked something. It usually took two or three tries before we acquired a taste for a particular plant, but eventually the plant became part of our diet.

Medicinal Another cough medicine Grandfather used to use was made from primrose. He would take a small palmful of crushed dry leaves and add it to one-half cup of hot water. It was allowed to steep for fifteen minutes, then taken in one-quarter-cup dosages four times a day. For a slightly stronger medication, use fresh leaves instead of dry, and allow them to steep for five minutes. The dried leaf tea is also good for digestive disorders. I find that it is very soothing to an upset stomach and to the digestive process in general. Some octogenarian friends take primrose tea twice a week as a tonic to keep their digestive system working. Some of them swear that it keeps their minds clear. I could count that as stupid superstition but oddly enough, none of them are senile.

Sweet Goldenrod (*Solidago odora*)

Description   Goldenrod produces a showy, bloomlike cluster of small, yellow blossoms which bloom between July and October. It is a lover of dry open woods such as the Pine Barrens. It is also found along the fringe of old roadways. When crushed, the leaves produce a sweet, aniselike odor. The leaves are parallel-veined, slender, toothless, and smooth with tiny transparent dots when silhouetted by the sky. The plant ranges from Texas east to Florida and north along the eastern United States coast to New Hampshire and Vermont. It is also found in a small area from Oklahoma to Montana.

Personality   In the fall of the year, I stand on the back porch of my farm and look out over the alfalfa fields. There, floating on the edges of the green fields like a frame, are the misty borders of goldenrod. For years, people have tried to destroy our goldenrod brothers because of hay-fever. If they would only look beyond the pollen, they would discover a fascinating plant. To me, it is the herald of oncoming autumn, a haven for so many birds and animals, and a delicious food and medication. There is nothing more beautiful than a goldfinch perched on top of a goldenrod flower head. Their colors blend into a unified pattern, as if the bird were composed of flower and the flower of bird until there appears to be no separation.

When I was a child, goldenrod was always a source of wonder. It seemed that so many insects gathered about its crown, and odd-shaped exotic goldenrod spiders hid there. We watched as these spiders lay in wait for unsuspecting insects and proved masters of camouflage, patience, and predation. To us, the life of the goldenrod spider was one of the best. Not only did food come to him, but he had a clear view of everything that went on in the surrounding fields. Each goldenrod plant seemed to have its own spider protector, and he defended his turf vigorously.

Beneath the goldenrod groves was a network of animal trails; animals were protected from attack by the thickness, which was full of things edible. Under these goldenrod colonies there was always a life and death battle, mingled with the beauty of the showy tops. We couldn't understand why people never picked goldenrod or admired its beauty, for we thought it was one of the most beautiful flowers of the field. It was incredible to us that people would prejudice themselves to that beauty because someone else was allergic to the plant. It often seems that when one authority cautions against something, the disease of prejudice takes over all. Even if I did have hay fever,

I thought, it would not stop me from savoring the elegant beauty of this plant.

My first introduction to goldenrod was on a utilitarian level, and it probably saved my life, or at least was instrumental in keeping me from freezing to death. It was exceedingly cold and windy in the pinelands; winds whipped frigid, humid air right through the clothing, and the ground was covered with a deep, crusty snow. The skies looked forlorn and dark, heralding another upcoming storm, probably a frozen rain judging by the temperature. We tried desperately to make our camp. Debris for our huts didn't come easily and by the end of our building, we were soaked to the skin. Parts of our clothing had frozen on us, and we were sure that we were in the grip of hypothermia.

We had a suitable bow drill but no tinder. Most of the tinder that we would normally glean from the landscape was wet or frozen from the snow. Rick spied a patch of dead goldenrod growing near camp. Many of the heads were encrusted with ice and snow, but there were a few that looked dry and serviceable. We used the dried stalks to add to our fire as kindling, knowing that it would catch quickly and hold a flame long enough for the rest of the harder woods to catch. With frozen hands and trembling bodies, we began to gather the tops of the goldenrod, buffing them into a bundle so that they would become light, fluffy, and easily caught in the flame.

Feeling the cold begin to overtake our bodies to a point where we were losing muscle control, we began to pump the bow drill. Our feeble attempts finally began to produce not only smoke, but also a tiny coal. To our amazement, that tiny coal grew larger and larger in the goldenrod tinder bundle and quickly burst to flames. The intensity of the heat caused us to drop the bundle, but it tenaciously kept burning. It seemed a long time as we pushed the bundle across the snow and into the fire, but it persistently burned and finally gave us a glorious blaze. I always look to the misty yellow patches from that day on as the fire that once saved my life during a rather intense survival situation. An offering I shall never forget.

During the whole episode of the fire, Rick had received a bad burn as he tried to move the hot tinder bundle into the fire area. Again the goldenrod came to our rescue. Grandfather brewed a strong tea from the leaves that were left on the dead stalks and applied it cold to Rick's burns. The tea proved soothing to a point where the pain was taken away, never to return, the burn forgotten. That night we warmed ourselves even further by drinking the mild tea made from the tender goldenrod leaves gathered that summer. To this day, I call that campout the goldenrod weekend.

Food   Goldenrod tea is, by far, one of my favorite teas. The fresh or dried flowers and new leaves make an excellent anise-flavored tea, when steeped in hot water from ten to fifteen minutes. I also use the shredded green leaves, in small amounts, as an additive to wild salads or sprinkled on boiled cattail corms. The flowers can also be used as a garnish, but only when eaten in small amounts. One of my most favorite and very healthful tea mixtures combines equal parts of goldenrod tea with rose hip tea. Adding a mint tea also makes a dynamic brew.

Medicinal   Another time goldenrod came to my rescue was when I accidentally ran through a yellow-jacket nest. I had been stung repeatedly on the face until it was twice normal size. Nothing seemed to relieve the swelling or pain until Grandfather used the powers of goldenrod to help me out. He first made a lotion from the flowers by boiling them in one cup of hot water, straining, then mixing the liquid with tallow. The lotion was then applied to the bites. On top of each sting, he placed a poultice of chewed leaves. The swelling went down quite quickly and the pain disappeared almost immediately.

Another use of goldenrod is as an all-around tonic and health drink. A palmful of flowers are added to one cup of hot water and simmered for one-half hour. The old-timers take one-half cup a day, every other day. Stronger teas can be made by also combining the green or dried older leaves. Use of the older leaves makes the drink a little bitter. A stronger and more bitter tea made exclusively from the older leaves can be used as a mouthwash or a general skin wash. The tonic tea is also very good in the aid of digestion and to minimize gas.

Greenbrier (*Smilax rotundifolia*)

Description   Greenbrier is a climber, using tendrils, and sporting beautiful parallel-veined leaves. They intertwine into beautiful viny patches, sporting tenaciously sharp thorns. The flowers are tiny and green, and the berries small. The greenbrier species can be found in a multitude of locations, from damp woods, thickets, bottomlands, and swamps. It blooms in mid-summer and bears fruit in late fall. Some southern species retain their leaves throughout the year. It is found in the southern United States from eastern Texas to Florida, and north into Maine and adjacent Canada. It also can be found in central United States from Montana to Oklahoma.

Personality   Of all the plants that are intriguing to me, the most by far is the greenbrier. It is a plant that demands respect, from its rough tangle of near-impenetrable growth to its needlelike stickers. The greenbrier itself is fascinating, but even more so is the protection it provides for so many animals. To them it provides more than adequate cover from predation and makes it almost impossible for any of the larger predators to penetrate its confines. In parts of the Pine Barrens, it grows so thick that travel through it is possible only by crawling carefully on your belly along the tiny animal runs that crisscross the patches. In certain areas, it could take days just to travel a few hundred yards.

The brier patches and I are old friends or old enemies, depending on how fast I choose to travel through them. To me they are a source of wonder, excitement, and the most bizarre forms of exploration. When I was a boy, I used to spend hours carefully crawling through the tangles, viewing the animal highways, hideaways, feeding areas, bedding areas, and protection areas. Whole communities of animals called these patches home: raccoon, rabbit, grouse, pheasant, and many others. It wasn't uncommon to find a good-sized deer curled up in a small open area beneath the thicker tangles. It would leave me scratching my head with wonder on how he ever got in. Out of all the brush tangles, the brier patches were the most protective and impenetrable.

To a tracker and naturalist, it was a place you could truly say had never before been explored by any man. It was littered with the daily life-and-death struggles that went on all the time. If a boy was good at concealing himself, he could also use the briers to his advantage and watch the grand shows that transpired along the road network, completely unobserved by the animals. The ground was littered with feathers, bones, feeding signs, and so many other things. Just ten feet of trail would keep me busy for many hours in thorough exploration.

I also learned from the animals and birds who inhabited the brier patches. When we were camping in wild-dog areas, we took a page out of the animal books and built our debris huts in the center of the more impenetrable brier patches so that the dogs could not get through easily. Many times I've escaped injury by diving down one of the brier trails to avoid the marauding dogs. The more time I spent in the confines of the briers, the more they became a second home. With years of practice, I could move through even the most inscrutable places with great ease and without getting stuck. The security I felt in the confines of these brier jungles was beyond description; it was always a safe haven.

One huge brier patch, in particular, housed one of our permanent camps. To get to the camp area, one had to know the tricky maze of trails that led to a large open area just off center of the patch. The camp area had a thick canopy of brier, except for a small opening over our campfire area. A double-debris hut was located at one end, and numerous backrests, small hide racks, and cache areas were located throughout. It was a place where we found the ultimate security; so secretive and camouflaged was the whole camp that hunters would pass right next to it without even suspecting, even if we had a fire going.

The animals that lived in the confines of the patch were never hunted and soon became our friends. After a while, they would pay us no notice and come right into our camp to beg for food. I guess they figured that nothing dangerous would ever venture into the briers so we were considered friends. Many of the smaller animals would sleep right with us and periodically a deer would enter the compound to take up residence during the hunting season. The brier might as well have been an isolated island where the animals were not used to man and found no danger in us. However, anytime we ventured outside the patch, we were considered dangerous and the animals would flee. I feel that it was an unwritten natural law that anything in the patch was automatically hiding from predators, and shared a common bond.

The brier patch was not only a source of protection and security, it also fed us periodically throughout the spring. When we were hungry and did not feel like venturing out into the outer world, we would nibble the succulent new tendrils. They were absolutely delicious and very filling. One could not help but feel even closer to the brier people when they added their gifts of food to their ultimate protection. We learned a valuable lesson with the brier people. If you looked deeper into them than just their rough, painful exterior, you could find a haven of tranquillity and security. Pain is what most people and predators see, and it prevents them from going any further.

The brier went far beyond protection and food uses, giving us a number of other utilitarian uses that were critical in survival situations. Many times the stout but supple stems provided us with cordage for binding. By braiding several strands together, we could produce a quick rope that would hold our weight. Many times we used the ropes to help us climb trees or cross streams. Stripped of thorns, the brier stems could also be woven into serviceable baskets and mats of superior quality. However, when the stems dried out, they would become brittle. Soaking in hot tallow retards this drying process to a point where a basket stays strong for decades. The dried stems also made great, volatile kindling, and the green thorns made great spur attachments for fish spears.

Food   Grandfather introduced us to even more fascinating uses of greenbrier. He knew of our greenbrier compound and was the first to tell us the new green tendrils were a delicious nibble. We loved the taste, but because of the treacherous personality of the plant, we figured that there was little else we could eat. Once, while camping in our compound, Grandfather returned with a bag of tendrils and new green leaves. As he simmered these in a container of water, he methodically munched on a few green leaves, which made us realize that the leaves could be eaten alone or added to flowers. The cooked greens he prepared were even more tasty and soon became one of our favorites.

One spring, Grandfather gathered some new shoots of greenbrier and steamed them as he would wild asparagus. These were even better than the cooked greenbrier greens, and later we found that they could also be nibbled raw. We were thrilled at all the uses of the greenbrier, and our respect and intrigue for this plant far surpassed its tenacious stickers. Later that summer we discovered more of the greenbrier's edibility. The roots could be broken up in cold water and the powder allowed to settle to the bottom. The fibers were removed, the water poured off, and more water added as a washing process. After the sediment settled, the washing procedure was repeated. The rich red powder was then dried for future use.

One small palmful of the powder mixed with one cup of boiling water produced a fine gelatin. This gelatin could be mixed fifty-fifty with any natural flour and used as a soup thickener. It could also be added to cold water sweetened with honey, and used as a cold refreshing drink. One of my favorite teas is made by taking cold greenbrier root drink and mixing fifty-fifty with a hot mint tea. Sumac-ade can also be mixed with the greenbrier drink for an outstanding healthful taste.

Medicinal I once had a severe second-degree burn which Grandfather treated with cool gelatin made from the root of greenbrier. He mixed the gelatin with tallow and applied as a salve. He has also used the gelatin and tallow mixture for other skin abrasions, after adding one-third tannic acid boiled from acorn husks. This I found to be very soothing, healing the abrasion quickly. I do not suggest that the ointment be placed on large open wounds, as it may cover an infection. Chewing the fresh leaves, then soaking them in strong tannic acid tea from acorn boilings make a great poultice to relieve the itch of chigger and red-ant bites.

Greenbrier is a dynamic plant with so many uses. It is truly a grand brother of survival situations. We learn quickly that even though the plant can inflict pain to the careless and is not particularly beautiful, it still has a myriad of helping properties if we can only learn to look beyond the superficial. Greenbrier was a plant that taught us to look beyond physical appearances to find the loving spiritual beauty beneath. So, too, with all entities of Creation.

Hemlock Tree (*Tsuga canadensis*)

Description Hemlock is a lover of hilly and rocky woods. It looks irregular and feathery from a distance. The cones are small and medium brown. The leaves are white underneath and in flat sprays. The bark is dark and rough. The needles are attached by slender stalks, and the twigs are rough when the leaves are removed. Hemlock grows from Canada southward to Indiana and Maryland. Following the higher mountain elevations, it can reach into Georgia.

Personality It was our first trip out of the Pine Barrens, and Rick and I had been excited about it for weeks. Our parents were going to let us camp in a Boy Scout camp area in upstate New York all by ourselves. The beauty of it all was that the camp was not in use at this time, but since my dad was the scout master, we had special permission. It was our first real excursion to the mountains, and we looked forward to fishing in the lakes, playing in the waterfalls, exploring the ridges, and most of all, learning all about the new things we hoped to encounter. We packed more identification manuals and collecting equipment than we had camping equipment, but we felt that creature comforts had to give way to more important things.

We were dropped off on Friday, with no real restrictions other than to stay out of trouble and have fun. We did have one responsibility to Grandfather in that we had to collect the bark and greens of the hemlock tree for his medicine bag. Just the thought of collecting those things for him uplifted our spirits and made us feel like important herbalists. Our first order of business, however, was to have fun. We began exploring the upper ridges, then the waterfalls. We fished for hours on the deserted lake and made a beautiful camp in one of the lean-tos. We had a feeling of ancient explorers, unencumbered by any time schedules or commitments.

The Hemlock trees, which Grandfather spoke of, were all around the camp area, but he wanted the parts from a small one, preferably growing near a stream or waterfall. To him, the area in which a plant grew affected the potency and worth of its medicinal value. Hemlock collected from the banks of a stream was very soothing, while that collected from a high ridge was very powerful, and hemlock collected from the damper areas was a little of both. So our last day we dedicated to locating absolutely the best tree possible, collecting in a very reverent and spiritual manner.

We collected the parts of the tree in a very careful and sacred way, taking care not to damage the tree or retard its growth. For many hours we prayed and meditated over the little tree, collecting its parts very slowly and methodically. Little did we know that we were being watched from far up in the canyon by an old man who lived in the hills. He was delighted to watch our collection and must have realized that we had been trained by one of the ancients. As we started up the canyon and back to camp, we were startled to see him standing there, wrapped in skins, appearing a cross between an old mountain man and a Native American.

He told us that he was very intrigued by our collecting methods and that he suspected that we had been trained by someone very important. He was also very interested in hearing our story, so we accepted his invitation to go back to his cabin for a cup of tea. His cabin was old and nearly dilapidated; old furs hung on the wall, his possessions few. We sat down in his room in front of an old stove and were mesmerized by his large and varied store of bottled herbs and bunches of drying plants hanging from the rafters. A short conversation revealed that he was a hermit, but he made his money treating the old farmers of the area with his widely known herbal remedies.

We stayed for hours, listening to his stories and he to ours. He was thrilled that there were some young people left who were intersted in the powers of the ancient herbal remedies. He introduced us to the hemlock tree by allowing us to savor some freshly brewed tea made from its leaves, and his bread was made partially from dried inner bark of the large hemlocks. We were utterly captivated by his stories, especially the fact that he was part Native American and had lived for nearly thirty years in those hills. He literally lived off the land, making all of his own things, remaining quite happy with his life-style. In the hours we spent with him, we learned a great deal about the philosophy he lived by, which was not too different than Stalking Wolf's.

Our notebooks and minds were crammed with his flow of information. He spoke of ancient hunting methods and how to make the weapons, how to stalk, how to live in balance with the forest, and how to communicate with all things. Here was another man that was very much like Grandfather, with the same philosophy that he learned solely from the forests. He had no books and no human teachers, only nature's university to guide him along his path. We were in awe, for only in Grandfather had we noticed a man of such inner peace, love, and joy, living in a totally balanced harmony with the Earth. Our parting produced tears and heartbreak, but he assured us that we would meet again because the people of the Earth have the same spirit, and there is no separation. Time, distance, and space are not factors in keeping those of like heart apart.

Months later, we visited Grandfather in his northern camp. Out of the shelter walked our old friend from the northern woods. Our hearts soared with the eagles, as we found that he was to spend the summer helping Grandfather teach us. To this day, I do not know how he found Grandfather or how Grandfather found him. All we knew was that those two seemed to have known each other for decades and spoke a common tongue. For us, it was one of the most fascinating summers we ever spent. Our knowledge of woodlore increased, and our spirits began to assimilate and bring to reality the spirit of communication.

Food   Certainly, it was the old man of the north woods, who we called Hemlock Medicine, who introduced us to the uses of hemlock. Through him and Grandfather, we learned so much more about this very powerful tree. Its leaves could be steeped in hot water for one-half hour to produce a very healthful and delicious tea. Mixed with mint or pine-needle tea, it made an even more delicious drink. The inner bark of the hemlock tree could be removed, dried, and pounded into flour. The flour could be used as a soup thickener or added to other natural flours to make a great bread, especially when made into ash cakes. Many people find the inner bark a little distasteful, but it is an acquired taste, and with repeated use you will find it rather delicious.

Medicinal   Grandfather used to make a tea from the inner bark of new twigs. A palmful of inner bark simmered for ten minutes in two cups of water and strained would make a very powerful medication with many uses. It could be used as a mouthwash or a toothpaste for swollen gums. One-half cup taken over the course of a day would settle stomachs and clear up diarrhea. A stronger tea would make a good skin wash and antiseptic for all sorts of sores, abrasions, and stings. It even worked well on sunburn and poison ivy. The powdered bark could also be sprinkled in the shoes to cut down on the discomfort of sweaty, tender feet. In addition, it also effectively cuts down on foot odor. Before stalking, some people also apply it to the underarms and groin to cut down on human odor.

Jewelweed (*Impatiens pallida*)

Description   The jewelweed stems are succulent, transparent, and very watery. The leaves appear silvery when placed under water. The flowers are pale yellow, closed at the larger end, horn shaped, and spotted. The yellow flowers bloom from July to October. Jewelweed is a lover of the wet, shady places ranging throughout most of the Appalachian range south to Georgia, and into Kansas and Montana.

Personality   Another name for jewelweed is "spotted touch-me-not." Our first encounter with this beautiful and helpful plant was as a game. We had been exploring a swamp area in the northern pine barrens where the hardwood forests and swamps took over, and we came upon this exotic-looking plant by chance. We admired its urn-shaped flowers, looking as if they came from a distant jungle area, blending beautifully with their stems that looked like they were more composed of water rather than stem. We closely observed the little flowers for hours until finally I reached out and gently touched one of them. It popped from its seat, almost magically, and shot several inches away. We were shocked by the whole process.

The remainder of the day was spent trying to decide why certain flowers did the jumping while others remained stationary. What survival value could this jumping effect have? Upon closer inspection, the ripe seeds seemed to jump even more than the flowers, propelling themselves far and wide. The plant was very intriguing to say the least. Even the stems looked transparent so that we could see the bundles clearly growing within. Plants like this held us in awe and curiosity to a point where we would not be satisfied until we learned everything about them.

It was a few weeks later that I was to learn of the more practical values of the jewelweed, other than the source of wonder. I had been trailing a rabbit for quite some time and inadvertently wandered through a large patch of poison ivy. Grandfather, fortunately, was looking on and had witnessed my lack of observation. Being dressed only in a loincloth made the situation worse. After tracking was over, he laughingly pointed to the trail I had left through the ivy and told me that I had better go to the river to wash off. I knew that too much time had elapsed since I first encountered the poison ivy, and all the washing in the world would not stave off the infection.

Grandfather met me at the stream holding a large bunch of jewelweed. I was astonished that he knew of the plant, but I had no idea what he was doing with it. He broke up the stems, without a word, and told me to rub it vigorously all over my body. Without question, I followed his directions while asking a myriad of questions as to why the plant seeds seemed to pop off. First things first I thought, and I would ask him about why I was using jewelweed as a wipe. Most things soon forgotten, I went about my daily routine, the poison ivy and jewelweed now far from my thoughts.

The next day I expected to awake covered with poison ivy, but there was not a trace. Ecstatic that I would not have to suffer with any of the dreaded itch, I found Grandfather and asked him how I had avoided becoming affected. He then explained that jewelweed has rich acids in its stems and leaves that neutralize the effects of poison ivy. He also explained how it deadens the pain of nettle stings and can be used on many other skin maladies, especially those that itched. Upon my asking him how the plant got its name, we traveled to the river, where we submerged a leaf. Sure enough, when the leaf went under water, it sported a beautiful jewellike sheen, thus the name.

Food   Jewelweed sprouts make a delicious cooked green. They should be gathered before they reach six inches tall, and boiled from ten to fifteen minutes in two changes of water. It is not good to use the water for drinking as it can be mildly poisonous. It does, however, make an excellent skin wash. My first memorable taste of jewelweed green was during an exploration hike when Grandfather cooked a batch up and served them with cattail corms. It made a delicious dish, one I will never forget, and now frequently feed to my family.

Medicinal   The medicinal values of jewelweed have been mentioned above. The crushed stems and leaves can be wiped onto affected areas from poison ivy or nettle sting to minimize or take away the symptoms. I find that it also works well on bee and other insect stings, sunburn, abrasions, and blisters. I find that some of my students use jewelweed squeezings as a remedy for acne and other blemishes with good results.

The juice from the cooked green makes an all-around skin wash, especially during survival situations where the lack of water makes bathing impossible. It effectively cleans out all minor cuts and prevents infection when they can't be washed with natural soap and water. I make an insecticide by mixing jewelweed juice fifty-fifty with the tannic acid boilings of cedar bark. Wiped on the legs, face, and arms, it seems to keep ticks away. I also keep a vial of the juices in my survival camp, in case I need some quick remedy for poison ivy into which I have inadvertently wandered. I make mud for removing bee stingers by mixing the juice of jewelweed with mud. Not only does it soothe the sore and remove the stinger, but it cuts down on the unpleasant burning. Mixing jewelweed juice with tallow also makes a good poison-ivy ointment for extremely itchy areas.

Milkweed (*Asclepias syriaca*)

Description Milkweed is a lover of abandoned fields and roadsides, especially in dry soil. It is a beautiful plant, hairy, erect, and a gray-green. It is usually unbranched. Seed pods are tear-drop shaped, pointed, and very warty in appearance. The flowerheads are in beautiful, slightly drooping, domed arrangements. They bloom all summer in pastel colors—white, buff, and dull purple. Milkweed is found in Canada, south to Georgia and Tennessee, and west into Kansas and Iowa.

Personality Gathering dried milkweed stalks in late fall for cordage always turned into a fun-filled adventure. We picked a day that was bright and sunny and filled with mild but gusty wind—a day we were sure that the milkweed skeletons were turning from green to gray. This graying color was the best indicator of the finest cordage, especially when it was meant for leaders on our fishing lines. Gathering consisted of cutting the old stems, stripping the old leaves, and scattering the parachutelike downy seeds. This seed sowing was usually done with the utmost artistic movements, which usually shifted rapidly into all-out wars.

We would usually gather the stems together in neat bundles and pile the partially opened seed pods in the center of the field. Once the gathering was complete, we would set about breaking open the pods and throwing the seed parachutes to the wind. It wasn't long before the entire field was turned into a war zone, resulting in Rick's and my being covered thoroughly with down. In the more raucous and violent wars, especially when one of us was losing, we would wrestle each other until one of us triumphantly stuffed milkweed down into the other's mouth. Sometimes these wars lasted for many hours, often involving muck, which brought back visions of the old tar-and-feathers punishment. I don't know how many people were frightened by two strange-looking fuzzy beings walking along the trails, but I suspect we were often mistaken for the Jersey Devil and his friend.

Years later, we would use what we had learned during our milkweed wars to scare people away from the Pine Barrens. As the four-wheel–drive craze began to take hold, local troublemakers would drive into the forest, cut down live trees for firewood, drink their beer, then throw their cans all over the forest. The Pine Barrens began to look like cancer had hit it, and we were helpless to do anything about it. A few times after losing our tempers, we would get beaten up by the marauders; at other times, they would purposely run through our camp areas and destroy our shelters.

One night, after a particularly muddy milkweed war, we were heading down to the swimming hole to wash off when we inadvertently passed one of these destructive parties in progress. We cautiously tried to pass by without anyone noticing, but someone caught our movements out of the corner of his eye. When he shouted, we thought that we were in for another beating, but the shouting quickly flowed into shrieking. Within moments, there were people running everywhere, diving for trucks, running down trails, and generally panicking. The whole area cleared of people within moments, and the Pine Barrens were left again to the night sounds. For the life of us, we couldn't figure out what had happened. At best, we thought that they believed the police were on their way.

The next day in school the story unfolded into all its glory. People talked of a beer party in the Pine Barrens where two ghostlike figures had appeared from the swamp. These creatures then miraculously disappeared back into the mist. After a while the story was blown out of all proportion to a point where the whole school believed that some hideous monster was lurking in the swamps, waiting to carry off anyone that came close. Rick and I were beside ourselves with delight, and we did what we could to perpetuate the story, even adding more to it until the whole affair became the frequent topic of conversation, especially to the people involved in beer parties.

We listened closely to conversation, waiting for clues as to where and when the next party would be held. By Thursday, we knew that the party would take place near Wells Mills at the far corner of the lake. We planned for hours just what we would do, where we would come from, and our escape. This had to be one of the best acts of terror that the pines had ever seen. To us, the whole future of the forests were at stake, and we saw our chance to put an end, once and for all, to the slaughter. Every detail was in place, every prop. We placed our camp on a hidden island in the swamp for a close escape.

The people began to gather at sunset, and by nightfall, the party was in full swing. As we mucked ourselves up, we could hear constant chopping, as trees fell and were fed to smoldering fires. The night was perfect, for the moon was nearly full and the clouds seemed to play tag with the stars. Mist gathered on the lake and grew thick around the swamps. We powdered ourselves with huge piles of milkweed down, which blended beautifully with the moonlight and the mist, making our outlines hazy and ghostlike. As we started to walk across the swamp, feral dogs began barking in the distance and the party grew strangely quiet.

Someone spotted us in the distance. Initial shrieks quieted quickly as everyone jumped to their feet and stood transfixed, gazing in sheer terror across the swamp. One girl screamed that the creatures were floating not walking. At that instant, as if planned by the Creator, a feral dog let out a bloodcurdling howl very close to the party camp. Instantly, in a frenzy of motion, people ran to their vehicles. Some tripped, others ran into trees, some even crashed into each other as they all tried to get out through one small trail. Screams slowly disappeared in the distance, and the rumble and clatter of the vehicles died away.

We spent the next day gathering up articles of clothing, axes, knives, shoes, and miscellaneous other things left behind by the party-goers. Ironically, there wasn't another beer party in that area of the pines for over two years. Years later, we would use our milkweed down again to drive more and more of the malignant beer parties from the forests. Even now, well into my thirties, I still partake in a little ghostly terrorism. I have to laugh at the way I found a utilitarian use of a plant that no one had ever dreamed of considering. It's a use that, in essence, affects the whole use of a forest area.

Food   We were told that the white, milky sap of milkweed was bitter and slightly poisonous, though it was a very effective medication. We were frightened by the prospects, especially the first time we ate the milkweed, hoping that the boiling process had, in fact, rendered the juices harmless. We were camped on the edge of an old abandoned field, one of the places we collected milkweed and dogbane shafts. Grandfather began to collect the small milkweed plants that were just a few inches tall. To add to our worry of the plant's milky poison, we were afraid that he would have a hard time telling the difference between the young milkweed and dogbane plants. The dogbane is very poisonous.

Grandfather sat us down by a small patch of the plants and pointed out that young milkweed has fuzzy leaves, while young dogbane is smooth. Butterfly weed also looks like young milkweed, but lacks the milky sap. Collecting should be done very carefully, especially since there are so many poisonous look-alikes. Grandfather was always extremely careful to teach us all the intimate details of plants so that there could be no mistake. Where people run into problems, even experienced herbalists, is often from not knowing the baby plants and not paying attention to small detail.

We gathered the baby plants and brought them back to camp. Grandfather boiled a small and a large pot of water. He placed the plants into the boiling water for about a minute, poured off the water, then poured in new boiling water from the other pan. He repeated the process two more times then boiled the plants one final time for about fifteen minutes more. We were curious as to why he did not add cold water to the next boiling process and why there were so many changes of water. He explained that to add cold water to the boiling process and reboil would only fix the bitterness. The frequent changes of water would also render the poisonous properties and bitterness inactive.

When the milkweed shoots were finally served up, we stared at them for quite a long time. Our fear of the poison or the mixup with the dogbane was foremost on our minds. Grandfather had finished his and was still walking, so we decided to try it. After all, he had never done anything to hurt us before. The plants were absolutely delicious, though the first swallow was quite difficult. Later, we found that the flower buds, the young pods, and the tiny top leaves could be eaten in the same way. These were equally delicious.

Grandmother showed us another delicious part of the milkweed plant. She gathered the flowering tops, boiled them for a few minutes in two changes of water, dipped them in batter, and deep-fried them. They made a most delicious milkweed fritter. The flowers can also be added to ash-cake batter after being boiled in the same way. These also make a good meal and can be carried on long trips for a fast snack.

Medicinal For a few years I had a wart on the back of my thumb near the knuckle. Nothing I tried would ever take it away. Even having it burned off twice had no permanent results, as it kept coming back. I wouldn't have minded, but it interfered with my weaving and some of the other skills I had to perform where the back of the thumb was necessary. I eventually went to Grandfather and asked for his help. We walked to a milkweed patch, broke off a fresh stem, then placed a drop of the milk on my wart. He told me to do this twice a day for seven days then leave it alone. Within a week after the application, the wart dried up and disappeared. To this day, I have used it with limited success. It seems to work on some people but not others. It also seems to help clear up athlete's foot.

I also make a skin wash for poison ivy and other closed skin maladies by making a tea of the juice. I break up stems into cold water, strain, then use the whitish liquid as a wash for the feet. This is especially effective in hot weather when athlete's foot is prevalent.

I leave the lotion on for a few moments then wash off. I find that the water from the third boiling of the leaf-cooking process has a soothing effect on the digestive system. I take one-quarter cup just before bed.

Caution: *Milkweed sap can cause erratic heart beat.*

Mint (*Mentha spp.*)

Description   The mints are aromatic plants which have classic square stems and paired, toothed leaves. Their flowers, which bloom in violet, blue, red, or pink from mid-summer to early fall, have small lips that are clustered in terminal spikes. They are a lover of damp ground, wet meadows, and stream banks. One or more species can be found throughout the United States.

Personality   I came home one day carrying a plant that I had found near an old farm house that stood near one of our trails. I had no idea what the plant was or what it could be used for. All I knew was that it smelled good. The only smell I knew that came close to the smell of this plant was from a gum that my little brother Jim would chew once in a while. I planted the little plant in one of my mother's gardens, hoping that when Grandfather returned from his journey, I would have it at close hand and ask him about it. For a few weeks I watched that plant grow, sending up more shoots and growing fuller. Every morning before I left for school, I would spend a little time with it as if it were one of my children.

Near the end of the school year with its continuous warm weather, my mother began her gardening. She was always a loving gardener and never liked the thought of pulling weeds, but giving into the pressures of the neighborhood, she kept neat gardens. I remember coming home on the last day of school and seeing my mother in the garden with a huge pile of weeds beside her. My plant was in the part of the garden that she had just finished weeding, and I just knew that it would be some place in that batch of dying weeds. Horrified, I approached my mom and sheepishly asked her about my plant, as I looked over at the place it had been. I told her the story of the plant and how I had watched it grow, hoping that Grandfather could tell me more about it.

She smiled up at me and told me that my little plant was in good hands and that she would show me what it could be used for. She led me around to the sunny side of the house and there in a small garden all its own stood my little plant, healthier and bigger than ever. I was amazed that my mother had the forethought not to destroy the plant. I thanked her for not throwing away my plant, but I was curious to know how she knew that I had planted it. As it turned out, she did not know it was my plant, but because it was a mint plant, she wanted to cultivate it on her own because it could be used for food and flavoring.

139

I was beside myself with delight. I could not believe that my own mom knew about a wild plant, and what was even better, she was going to teach me all about it. I never realized how much she knew about the wild plants, and until this time I didn't think that she was the least bit interested. We went into the house and she brewed up two glasses of iced tea, took a few leaves from the mint plant, crushed them, then added them to the tea. The drink was absolutely delicious with the essence of the mint to give it a certain power and refreshing flavor. Later as we sat by the garden, she took a small piece of leaf and placed it on my tongue telling me not to chew or swallow it but let the flavor fill my mouth. It was more refreshing than the iced tea and felt wonderfully soothing to the mouth and throat.

I was amazed at my mother's love of mint. All summer long we nurtured our plant, watching it grow and spread through the whole garden. It was our unplanned project and we worked on it together quite often. The mint was responsible for showing me a new side of my mother I never knew, and we grew closer than we ever had before. By the following summer, our one mint plant had taken over the entire garden, and we had to weed some out so that the mint plants did not choke themselves or the other plants. We hung these weedings from the rafters of the kitchen and allowed them to dry. Mom would use them to make a tea or add to other teas to brew some delicious tea mixtures. She also used the fresh or dried leaves in many of her other recipes, especially her lemon meringue pies.

The first time I ever saw the mint plant used as a medicine was when one of the local children began to run a high fever. Grandmother was summoned to their deep woods farm to take care of the child, and she asked me to come along. Immediately realizing that the child's fever had to come down, she sent me running back to my house to collect a few handfuls of mint. She took the mint and added the leaves, stems, and flowers to boiling water and allowed them to steep for about twenty minutes, producing a strong tea. She cooled the tea, then wiped it over the feverish child. The fever broke and came down within a quarter hour.

Grandmother explained to me that the tea had a refrigerant property that helps cool the body in times of fever. Some mild tea was then brewed to help the little child sleep. Grandmother viewed the mint and all its relatives as very powerful medicines and had a high respect for the plants' medicinal properties. She rarely would use the plant as food or flavoring, though every once in a while, she would brew a strong tea and drink it for tonic properties or when her insides were a little upset. This, however, did not stop me from drinking my mother's tea mixtures; they were just too delicious to pass up and my mom was very healthy. I attribute much of her good health back then to the tonic values of the mint teas.

Food The green or dried leaves of mint can be used to brew a delicious tea. Steep the green or dried leaves in water from ten to fifteen minutes, longer if a stronger tea is desired, sweetened to taste if you prefer, and sip as you would any tea. The tea is delicious hot or cold, and I find it especially refreshing during the hotter summer months. Be careful, however, because the tea can be a strong medicine, having tonic and relaxing qualities similar to catnip.

The dried or green leaves can be used as a seasoning in many foods, giving them a delicious taste. I think it adds the essence of the wild to otherwise mundane dishes. I prepare the leaves for drying by hanging them upside-down from the rafters in a cooler section of my home or shelter. When thoroughly dried, I grind up the leaves into a coarse powder if it is to be used as a seasoning, or just break them up into small flakes if it is going to be used for a tea. Generally, the stronger teas and seasonings are made from the older healthy leaves. Milder teas and seasonings can be made from the younger succulent leaves. Milder still are the leaves gathered during the times that the plant is in flower.

Medicinal The medicinal qualities of mint are endless. One of the more esoteric medicinal qualities I discovered accidentally is what I call "rapture medication." Rapture medication can be obtained anytime I get stressed or fatigued, especially during hot summer days. I simply find a huge patch of mint, crawl into it, and lie down and relax. Especially on warm windless summer days, the body seems to sink into the Earth and become one with it. You can't tell where your skin ends and the Earth begins, there is no inner or outer dimension. The upper body, especially the nose, is bathed in the thick intoxicating fragrance of the plant, and you drift off into endless relaxed bliss, totally removed from all outside stresses. It is as if you are in a mint temple, close to the mothering power of the Earth. During the winter months, I collect small bags of dried mint to use as sniffers. Anytime I miss summer, I just reach into my drawer, pull out the bag of mint, and take a deep sniff. This immediately propels me back to the reverie of the mint temples.

All members of the mint family have similar characteristics. A strong tea can be brewed from the leaves collected on a hot sunny day, preferably before flowering time. These leaves can be dried or used fresh, the dried leaves producing a weaker tea. Brew the tea by steeping a large palmful of leaves in a pint of water. Steep from fifteen to thirty minutes and allow to cool. The tea can be wiped externally onto the body to help bring down fever or to be used to alleviate skin pain. A cooling bath can be made by adding one quart of strong tea to warm bath water.

A mild tea made by steeping a small palmful of leaves in one cup of water for fifteen minutes can be used for many ailments. First, it makes a good all-around tonic drink for health, and can be used as a mild sedative for nervous headache, migraine, and general nervousness. The same tea has cough suppressant capabilities and alleviates cramps, heartburn, abdominal pains, upset stomach, and especially insomnia. I do not suggest the use of very strong teas for internal problems, as the prolonged use may cause heart problems. At the most, take only one to two cups a day, but for no more than four days. Continue the dosage only after waiting at least seven days. I have found that a strong tea made from the flowers, stems, and leaves of the fresh plant are great for itching skin due to poison ivy, when used in a bath two to three times a week until the condition subsides.

Note: Gathering plants in their maturity makes stronger medicinals—experiment with various growth stages.

Red Mulberry (*Morus rubra*)

Description   Red mulberry loves rich soils and open woods, especially old farm areas. The leaves are finely toothed, sandy above and hairy below. They can have two or three lobes. The twigs are hairless and contain a milky sap. The bark is a beautiful reddish brown with smooth ridges. The fruit is pendantlike, red at first but becoming a deep purple when ripe. The fruit can be gathered in early summer. Red mulberry is found from Florida to Texas, north to New York, and also from Minnesota to South Dakota.

Personality   It was Grandmother who first taught me one use of the mulberry shrub. She was on her way on a gathering hike up north when I met her on the trail. I always loved to walk along with her and help with anything she was doing because she always told stories and taught me new things. No matter what I was doing, there was always time for a walk with her or, for that matter, any older person. This day was no exception, and as we walked, the stories flowed. She would point to a flower or plant and reminisce about when she was young, how she learned about that plant, and what it could be used for. In survival situations or living far from any doctor or pharmacy, folks had to learn to take care of themselves. Thus the old remedies became a way of life.

Grandmother was on her way to a huge mulberry patch that grew near an old abandoned farmhouse. She said I could help her dig the newer plants' roots, which she would powder and make into a laxative for her patients. We dug for hours, collecting the choicest roots, still making sure that the conservation of the plants were kept in mind. During the whole process, I was eating the mulberries, not noticing whether they were ripe or not, a common fault among young boys. This continued for hours as I got lost in Grandmother's stories and the methodic collecting of roots.

When I finally got up off my knees and began to walk home, I felt strangely sick and dizzy. The landscape felt as if it were made of liquid and I was a small boat. Everything was moving up and down. Animal and bird voices sounded strange and mystical. I felt disoriented and forgot where I was and where I was going. Out of the corner of my eye I began to see things move; shadows became animated, and colors strange. The sickness continued until I fell to the ground vomiting, yet laughing at the overall hilarity of the situation. The condition worsened and I began to tremble, feeling paranoid and extremely nervous. I mistook every rustle of the brush for

143

a wild dog, and my imagination began to run wild.

Grandmother knew instantly what I had done and helped me slowly back to her house. I did not know that the unripe berries can cause violent upset stomach and nervousness. Nor did I realize that they also contained hallucinogens. Nevertheless, I was sick and not getting any better. Grandmother put me to bed and gave me a cup of mullein flower tea to settle my stomach and calm my nerves. I awoke the next morning with Grandfather, Rick, and Grandmother sitting around the bed, waiting and watching. My vision slowly cleared, but my head pounded very badly; my stomach still remained very queasy, and I felt weak. Another day slipped by as I drifted in and out of pain and sleep.

The following day I felt much better. The events of the past few days seemed like a distant nightmare, fuzzy memories at best, as if they never happened in reality. Grandmother was in the garden at her drying racks. The roots we had collected two days before were now dry. Lovingly, she scraped the bark from the root using a knife held at a right angle, a procedure which produced a coarse granular dust. This dust she would use for effective treatment of constipation in her patients or for herself. I helped her out but had to be filled in completely as to what had happened to me. The disorientation was still with me, and I felt as if I had lost two days of my life.

She did not explain the hallucinatory effects of the berries and green bark of the tree in terms of modern science. Instead, she took the old approach and spoke to me on a spiritual level, using ancient stories to explain the lesson. She told me that I had defiled the spirit of the bush by eating most of its fruit and not leaving anything for the other creatures to eat. The mulberry was punishing me for being greedy and not paying attention to what I was doing. She said that I had probably thanked the tree for the roots but failed to thank it for its berries. The bush was a guardian that taught people about greed and inattention.

Needless to say, I had a mighty respect for that bush. It took a long time before I would ever eat another mulberry, no matter how it was prepared. Even once when I was extremely constipated, I turned down Grandmother's remedy because I knew that it was made from the root bark of the guardian plant, and I didn't want to take the chance that it might still be mad at me. Grandfather and Rick would eat the new shoots of the mulberry in the spring and early summer. No matter how much I wanted to taste them, I just couldn't take the chance. It wasn't until I was older and understood what hallucinogens were that I finally began to eat mulberry again, and we became good friends. I still suspect the bush may yet be mad at me, however, so I always go out of my way to thank it and take very little from it when collecting.

Food The ripe berries of the red mulberry tree are delicious raw, but the berries from the white mulberry tree are usually too sweet to be eaten that way. White mulberries are best eaten dried and mixed with breads or muffins. They must be dried quickly in the hot sun so that they do not spoil. Red mulberries can be eaten raw, made into jelly, or cooked in pies and muffins. Crushed red mulberries, added to a little water and strained, make a delicious juice.

The new shoots of the mulberry, collected before the leaves erupt, are delicious. The shoots should be boiled in water for twenty minutes to one-half hour. Some old-timers like to change the water once during this process, but the water must be transferred hot. Please be conservative when collecting the shoots of mulberry or any other plant to insure future generations.

Warning: *The unripe berries, bark, and raw shoots contain hallucinogens which can cause extreme upset stomach and nervousness.*

Medicinal The old-timers used the bark of the mulberry root as a remedy for tapeworm. There are, however, better remedies for this ailment, and modern drugs should be used whenever possible unless you can't get to civilization. The powdered rootbark of mulberry is also a good laxative but should not be used in excess. For persistent constipation, change your diet and do not rely on mulberry for more than a day. Prepare the laxative by taking a small palmful of powdered rootbark and mixing it with a cup of warm water once a day. I do not recommend this for the novice.

Mullein (*Verbascum thapsus*)

Description   Mullein loves the dry waste places, old fields, and roadsides. Its first year, it produces a rosette of beautiful downy leaves. The second year a flowerstalk erupts, topped by a cylindrical flowerhead bearing beautiful yellow flowers. The leaves are large and quite soft, feeling much like velvet. Mullein is found throughout the United States.

Personality   The collecting of tobacco and tobacco mixes was one of the most sacred acts Grandfather, Rick, and I would undertake. Grandfather planted his own tobacco from the seeds passed on through generations of plants his people had once used. In fact, he had collected a myriad of tobacco seeds from all over the country, his favorite being that of the Seneca people. His tobacco was very sacred to him, and he tended the little patches he planted all over the Pine Barrens. To this day, some of the patches still grow year after year, reseeding themselves naturally. Always it was with the most tender care that he watched over his crop, sometimes even moving soil from other areas into his tobacco gardens.

Grandfather's tobacco was used for personal smoking, to make offerings, and to smoke in the Sacred Pipe, the People's Pipe. It was one of the most sacred herbs, for in its smoke were carried the prayers. It was given to the Native Americans by the Creator, and as with all plants, it was cared for as if it were a person, equal to ourselves. Most of the time the tobacco smoked was pure, especially in ceremony, but there were many mixes of the tobacco with other natural herbs, depending on the occasion and situation. There were smoking mixtures used for medication, for the sweatlodge, and for private use. Each mixture was meticulously collected, dried, prepared, and blended. Each step was lavished with prayer, meditation, and song. It was during the collection of the mixing ingredients that I was introduced to the powerful mullein people.

Before we ever knew the mullein as a medicine, utilitarian, tobacco additive, or edible plant, we were fascinated by its strange appearance. It loved the old farm fields and open places. Growing straight and tall as if shot from the heart of the Earth like a firework, it left in its trail a spray of soft velvety leaves. Its flowerheads were magnificent yellow spears of fiery color, splashed across the greenery of the fields. In our eyes, the mullein looked like people standing erect in the fields, worshiping the Creator. On days of patchy morning

146

mist, they stood alone and solitary, adding even more of a mystery.

Our first introduction to mullein was not medicinal, edible, or as a tobacco. Rather, we began to learn its utilitarian applications first. The learning of the most primitive use of the mullein came one late fall night as we sat around a campfire trying to work on our quillwork bags. The low flickering light of the campfire made close work difficult at best, and we struggled for hours trying to complete even the smallest sections. Grandfather, seeing our dilemma, cut a dried mullein stalk from a nearby field, then soaked the pocked flowerhead skeleton in a warm vat of tallow. He let it dry for a while then lit it, producing a marvelous torch that, to our amazement, lit the area extremely well.

Our next lesson in the uses of mullein came sometime later during a mid-winter campout. We had set camp and were searching the area for suitable wood from which to make our bow-drill fire apparatus. The bow drill is one of the ancient but dependable fire-making devices used for centuries. It is simply a spindle of wood spun hard against another flat, notched piece of wood, producing friction. Coals are formed in a notch, then blown to flames using a tinder bundle made from light bark and grass fibers. The process of making the bow drill takes some time to complete, and sometimes the gathering of the right wood that is dry enough can consume hours of searching.

Grandfather harvested a long straight mullein stalk from the field and gathered a dry limb from the nearby woods. He broke loose a flat section, notched the flat wood and abraded a rounded tip on the fat end of the mullein stalk, then cleaned the entire stalk of bumps and old dry leaves. By spinning the stalk between his palms with a back-and-forth motion and pushing down, he created on the fireboard the same smoking friction of the bow drill. The result was a very quickly made apparatus and fire. It took so little effort that we spent the next few months learning this hand-drill technique. Through experimentation with all the woods, we found that mullein was still the best for the hand-drill fires.

Our lessons with the mullein people were hardly over. In the weeks that followed, colds and flu began to run wild in our schools. Both Rick and I became afflicted with the usual cough and congestion, and felt utterly miserable. As our colds began to clear up, we went back to camping in the woods but with the usual discomfort of runny noses and congestion that seems to linger on and on. Grandfather took some dried mullein leaves from a small bag in his shelter and packed it into his personal pipe. We smoked the mixture, inhaling only a few times, as he instructed. He told us that mullein was a powerful medicine and that smoking the partially dried leaves would help clear up our congestion quickly.

The medication worked, the sniffles stopped, and we began to breathe much more freely. He told us that our medication was not finished, and we had to follow up the treatment with more mullein, taken in a different manner. We followed him to the field not far from the camp. He looked around the area at all the mullein skeletons that were sticking through the light cover of snow. It was as if he were looking for one in particular, and certainly he was. We were amazed when he brushed back the snow from a small south-facing slope, revealing a winter rosette of mullein leaves. We gathered only a few of the tiniest leaves from the center of the rosette then headed back to camp.

He boiled a small amount of water and added to it the broken mullein leaves. He covered the container, and we waited for a while until the top began to bounce around atop the pot. He then instructed us to deeply breathe in the vapors, filling our lungs. At first, our noses were stuffed and we could only pull the vapor through our mouths, but finally, all our air passages opened. Our persistent coughing also stopped, and we began to feel as if we never had colds. For the next two days we repeated the procedure twice a day and that was the last of our cold symptoms.

Unfortunately, too much of a good thing can be very dangerous and have a long-range effect on one's system. I began to abuse mullein whenever I had a cold, cough, or congestion. I used it sometimes when I didn't really have to. Sometimes I would use mullein so much that I would dangerously dry out all my nasal passages to an uncomfortable state. Because of all this abuse, I have developed an allergy of sorts to mullein. If I ever smoke or smell the vapors of the mullein plant, my nose begins to run and I get all the symptoms of a full-blown allergy. It no longer clears my head and opens my airways, but rather closes them up miserably. Needless to say, I learned my lesson that, like anything else, mullein should be used in moderation.

At certain times of the late summer we would go about the sacred business of gathering mullein for use as a tobacco additive. We would locate the small rosettes that had just taken hold. The rosette had to be perfect in shape, creating within itself a perfect sacred circle. From this, only the medium-sized leaves were gathered, a few from each plant, and they had to be absolutely perfectly shaped and unblemished. We then would dry the leaves in the late afternoon sun and bring them in every night and hang them upside-down in our shelter. For four days, we dried our sacred leaves for one hour of sun-drying a day, in just the right combination of sun and humidity. We finally hung them for the last time from the rafters of our shelters, fluffing them frequently for a week for even dryness.

The dried, dull green leaves were then carefully broken and placed in a large wooden bowl where they were kept for a few more days, stirred frequently again for even dryness. This mullein stash would be later mixed with tobacco and other herbs as needed. Sometimes the tobacco-mullein mix was kept already mixed, but most of the time it was mixed as needed. It was always important to remember that mullein had medicinal properties, so very little was used in any tobacco mixture and no mixture was ever fully inhaled.

Food   In early summer, as the mullein plants were rocketing toward the sun, but before the flower spikes developed, we would gather the uppermost leaves and dry them in bunches. These we would break up and drink as a delicious light tea. Stronger teas could be made by using older leaves that had been dried less, but we always had to remember that mullein had strong medicinal properties, and we would never drink more than a cup or two a day. In winter when all things were scarce or sleeping, we could brew a weak but warming tea from the few dried leaves found still clinging to the lower parts of the mullein skeletons. These were brewed much like Oriental teas, steeped in hot water up to one-half hour to extract the last remaining goodness of the plant's dried leaves.

Many times during a short break on one of our winter hikes, we would stop at a mullein patch. We would make our fire from mullein hand drills, boil water by using the mullein skeletons as fuel, and drink mullein tea. After our warm drink, we would smoke mullein-laced tobacco, then be on our way again, thankful for the power and versatility of this plant brother. In survival and at times of sickness, we would always find mullein a welcome friend.

Medicinal   I had been having trouble with a stomach virus for a number of days and had to be totally confined to the house, which was driving me nuts. Grandfather showed up in my room one afternoon with a flowering mullein spike, bearing his usual grin that said, "Why didn't you call me sooner?" He took a good handful of the flowers and steeped them in two cups of hot water, strained them, and gave me a full cup to drink. Immediately, my stomach cramps began to feel better, in fact, my whole digestive system was soothed by the warm tea. I felt mellow and tired within a few minutes and fell to sleep for fourteen hours, waking refreshed and feeling better. Mullein flowers make a good sedative for the head and digestive system. It also has a marvelous soothing effect on pain.

Another use of mullein as a medication is as a skin wash. Rick had a badly infected cut on his calf that would not heal. It began to look worse every day, and I knew that if it didn't heal, he would have to make a visit to the doctor. Grandfather had much to teach us about the new flowers that weekend, and he couldn't afford to have it delayed for another week. The flowers would have gone to seed. He boiled up some mullein leaves into a strong tea and washed Rick's wound. After rinsing, he crushed some dried leaves into a fine powder and placed it directly on the wound. That night Rick had a good sleep without the usual pain and swelling. The next morning the gash looked much better and showed signs of definite healing. The washing process was repeated and the wound powdered again. The cut cleared up normally.

The vapors from a strong fresh-leaf tea help clear congestion. Adding fresh flowers to the tea will increase the tea's potency. Smoking the partially dried leaves creates an even stronger dose, but should be used only as a last resort. Flowers can also be added fresh to this smoking mixture but only for very powerful decongestant properties. Use only once. The fresh flowers and leaves can be pounded and added to tallow as a skin balm for all sorts of skin problems. Mullein is one of the more powerful medicines and should be used sparingly and with the utmost respect.

I was horrified a few years ago when I heard a friend refer to the mullein as hunter's toilet paper. It could make a good toilet paper with its large soft velvety leaves, but I could never bring myself to use it in this manner. To me, the plant is all too sacred and I don't think this is a medicinal use. It is strange, but the same man who called it hunter's toilet paper developed a bad rash after he used it frequently during a bout of diarrhea. I look at it as poetic justice.

Black Mustard (*Brassica nigra*)

Description Mustard has a beautiful terminal cluster flower-head made up of small four-petaled yellow flowers. The lower leaves are very broad and deeply lobed. The seed pods point skyward, are slender, and end in a taper. They love waste grounds, old fields, and roadsides and can flower from spring to mid-fall. Mustard plants are found throughout the United States.

Personality Every spring there was a ritual that Grandpa Dandelion and I would perform. We would wander the old farm fields north of his home collecting wild mustard greens. Right after the first warm spell of spring, we would begin to comb the fields, gathering the newest and most tender leaves. These we would take back to his home and cook like spinach or add a little to salads. He cared for mustard almost as much as dandelion and would propagate it whenever possible. To him, cultivating the wild edible plants of the fields was done with the same meticulous care he used on his own gardens. He would guard these little patches zealously, and visit them frequently.

One of the best times for our mustard gathering was mid-spring. We would gather the unopened flowerheads and cook them like broccoli. It became one of my favorite wild foods, and I would look forward to those times of year when they were ripe for cooking. I felt like a wine producer watching his grapes until they reached the peak of flavor, then all at once collecting what he needed. In good years, the collecting season could go on for weeks, but we would never get tired of the greens. My parents enjoyed the mustard tops so much that they became a regular wild green at our table during the times of harvest. My dad especially enjoyed inviting over his friends to have them sample the vegetable, bragging about his boy who could find something edible even in a parking lot.

Grandpa Dandelion had as many uses for mustard as he did for his dandelion. To him, it wasn't only a delicious edible but a very powerful medication. Grandpa was the mustard supplier to all the herbalists of the area, and even Grandfather would use his powder for his own medicine bag. The preparation of the mustard powder was a careful process. We would spend hours collecting the seed pods, then more time extracting the seeds from the pods. He would collect the seed pods when they were still green, and age and dry them at home where he could easily harvest the seeds. The seeds were meticulously dried, finely ground, dried again, and stored in an earthenware container for future use.

The first time I ever saw the mustard powder used was when I was the patient. I was on my way back from a long, early spring hike and my feet were wet and cold. It was one of those times that I was wearing only light clothing and old tennis shoes riddled with holes, never expecting to travel very far from home, but ending up miles out of my way. I could barely walk by the time I reached Grandpa's back yard so I thought I would stop in and warm up. As I sat by the woodstove thawing out, my feet began to hurt and would not get warm. The longer I sat by the fire, the more pain I felt until I couldn't take anymore. I tried walking around but that only made my stiff joints feel worse and the skin burn.

Grandpa heated a large tub of water until it was slightly above body temperature. To this he added a little of the mustard powder and mixed it in thoroughly. He set it by the fire and told me to soak my feet in it for a while. It seemed to take forever to get my feet fully into the tub. The hot water seemed to be scalding even though I knew it was hardly warm. Once my feet were settled, however, they began to warm quickly and within minutes were back to normal. Now, I've had cold feet before and have soaked them in hot water but never with the quick results I got from Grandpa's mustard foot bath. Once the feet were warm, he told me to rinse off all the solution so that I would not get burned, explaining that mustard is very powerful and could cause irritation if left too long in place.

Since then I have seen mustard powder used for many things but always with the utmost caution. Everytime I witnessed Grandfather, Grandmother, or Grandpa Dandelion use mustard, it was always shrouded in warnings. I watched Grandpa prepare all types of wild mustard for medication powder but to him, the absolute best was the black mustard. This particular mustard, he said, was the purest and the most powerful, though to this day, I do not know why. Today I only use mustard as a foot bath for extremely cold feet, an appetite stimulant, or to reduce fever. My field tests have not proven the other treatments of mustard except on rare occasions, so I've all but abandoned them.

Food Grandfather was the first to give me my introduction to mustard during one of our summer outings. We had been camping for quite some time along one of our favorite fishing areas and subsequently had dined on fish for four days. On one occasion, we had fish for breakfast, and by that time, we were sick of it altogether. It wasn't so much the fish but how it was prepared and its blandness. Worse yet, we still had one fish left in our larder and it would be bad medicine not to use it. I strongly believe, as did Grandfather, that if we wasted the fish, it might be a long time until we ever caught another. The fish spirits do not take kindly to the waste of any life.

Grandfather, realizing that we had to eat another fish for dinner, took us on a hike a few miles from camp. There we collected the ripest mustard seed pods we could find and quickly headed back to camp. I had no idea what these strange seeds were going to be used for; I didn't even know that there was such a thing as wild mustard. Grandfather carefully cracked the pods and gathered a small pile of seeds. He ground these into a fine powder then mixed them with some tallow into a pasty substance. Without saying a word or answering any of our persistent questions, he put the paste in the larder.

Later that evening, we took the fish out to cook for dinner, and he heated the tallow and wiped it on the fish. As it cooked in the pan, he kept basting it with more of the tallow until the air was filled with the most delicious aroma. We ate the fish eagerly, now that it had a spicy taste that enlivened and transformed the taste of its flesh. Rick and I argued as to what the strange spice tasted like, for it was vaguely familiar to us. Finally, Grandfather could take no more and with a deep hoarse laugh slowly said, "M-u-s-t-a-r-d." We repeated this word several times before it dawned on us that he was talking about a common table condiment rather than some Apache spice.

Since then I have become an avid hot wild mustard maker. I gather the pods just before they become ripe and let them finish the process on my drying rack. I then extract the seeds and let them dry on my rack for several days and store them in a container until I make my mustard. Sometimes I will add the seeds directly to my pickling solutions for a hot wild taste to my pickles. To make my hot mustard, I grind the seeds into a fine powder and allow to dry for a few hours if I plan to store the powder for other uses. I then add wine or apple vinegar to the powder, just enough to make a thick paste. To this paste, I add water until it reaches the consistency of manufactured mustard. For those who prefer a different taste, leave the vinegar out. This method produces a very hot and spicy mustard; use it sparingly.

The new tiny green leaves gathered from the first rosettes of spring are great cooked like spinach. I prefer to change the water at least once, using preboiling water, and cook for a full ten minutes. The leaves will lose their bulk upon cooking so gather plenty, a few from each rosette. The new green leaves can also be chopped and a little added to wild salads. Though bitter if eaten alone, they even add a tang to otherwise drab salads. I also add the freshly chopped leaves and a little seed powder to Thousand Island salad dressing for a great wild spicy taste.

The flower tops can be gathered just before they erupt into bloom, and cooked like broccoli. They are best steam-cooked for five minutes but are also good boiled. They should not be cooked for more than five minutes, as they will lose their taste and become a little mushy. I make a great side dish by pouring melted cheese over the tops of the greens or just serving with butter. Some old-timers also use butter and lemon. The tender young seed pods, collected when the flowers are in the final stages of their bloom, are great added to salads. I also use them as a trailside nibble.

Medicinal When I cook new mustard greens, I always set aside some of the first waste water used for boiling. I store it in the refrigerator up to two days. I will reheat this tea until it is hot and use it to aid digestion. I find it works well when I am not feeling just right inside, and it seems to stimulate my appetite. I have also effectively used a poultice of older mustard leaves on a fresh insect bite with good results.

The fine-ground powder made from mustard seeds is the prime medicinal ingredient of mustard. I add a small palmful of powder to a pan of warm water to use as a foot bath, or add twice as much to your regular bath to help bring down a fever. All applications of mustard powder solution should be rinsed off after no more than five minutes of use because it can cause prolonged irritation. I am not in favor of mustard plasters as they can cause severe problems and burn the skin. Its medicinal value for arthritis and rheumatism does not prove out in my experimentation. I do not recommend mustard oil as it is extremely concentrated and has to be used with the utmost care. Only well trained herbalists should use this oil.

Stinging Nettle (*Urtica dioica*)

Description   Stinging nettle is an erect plant, usually unbranched. Its tiny hairs will sting and cause a rather bad rash, accompanied with tremendous pain. The plant has tiny green flowers and the leaves are paired and toothed. The nettle family inhabits many different soils, mostly waste grounds and disturbed soils. It is found from southeast Canada, south to West Virginia, and west to Minnesota, and also from New Mexico to Oregon.

Personality   I remember vividly my first intimate introduction to the nettles. I was swimming down at the old swimming hole on a particularly hot early summer day. I had been there most of the day, intermittently lying in the sun and cooling off in the water when the sun got too hot. By the end of the day, I was fiery red with sunburn and the pain was absolutely horrible. I was getting chills by the time the sun was setting. Putting on my clothes was not possible. Even the thought of clothing next to my skin made me hurt. I decided to run home in my bathing suit to prevent any undue pain, figuring that the walk would begin to warm me up.

I made a grave mistake by taking a short cut through an old farm field that had overgrown with hardwoods. I had never taken that route before, so I was unfamiliar with the territory. The waning light made me move along at a much quicker pace than I usually travel. Suddenly, my legs, stomach, back, and forearms felt as if they had been hit hard by a fireball. It was as if a thousand tiny bees were stinging me all at once, and the pain was only worsening instead of getting better. The pain was so bad I could hardly walk, and I thought I was surely going to die.

I abandoned my trip home and headed to Grandfather's camp, not only because it was closer, but I knew that if anyone could help me he could. I prayed that he would be there and have something that could help me out. I was sobbing when I approached the camp, and Grandfather knew instantly what had happened. Without a word, he ran back inside his shelter and reappeared with a greasy buckskin bag. The whitish ointment inside not only stopped the stinging, but it also soothed the sunburn almost instantly. He said that the ointment was very intricate to prepare but was essentially made of jewelweed, tannic acid, yarrow tea, tallow, and a few other ingredients. It was good for burns, bee stings, and nettle stings, from which I was suffering.

As the pain subsided and I was dressed again, we discussed

what had happened. First of all, I should have known better than to lie in the sun for such a long time. Secondly, I should have slowed down to a normal pace and been more cautious since I was going through new areas. And finally, I should have known about the nettle and respected its power. It was a very painful lesson, but I knew that the first thing I was going to do the next day was to retrace my steps and identify that damn plant, even if it was the last thing I ever did.

The next day, Grandfather and I went to the area where I took the short cut, and retraced my steps. It wasn't long before we found the accursed plant. I would have known that plant by myself for my tracks were quite obviously filled with pain just after I passed through the area. To my amazement, Grandfather carefully began to gather some of the smaller plants, grabbing them at the base and plucking them from the ground with his fingers. In astonishment, I asked him how he could touch those damn plants without getting stung and why the hell would he want to pick the little monsters. He simply said, "If you talk to them and show no fear, they won't sting." He also informed me that they were not little monsters but would soon be his supper.

At that moment, I thought that senility had finally taken hold of Grandfather, but I was intrigued by the way he could pluck them without getting stung. I swallowed my fear, spoke to the plants in a rather pleading voice, then grabbed one around the base as Grandfather had. Evidently, I must have shown some fear, for the little bugger bit me again. I walked back to camp thoroughly disgusted with myself but curious as to how Grandfather was going to eat these things. Surely, I thought, he must have a calloused mouth and innards, probably due to eating these things over a period of years. After all, I'd seen him eat some rather vile-looking, smelly, and tasteless things.

He took the nettles he had gathered and boiled them in a small amount of water for about fifteen minutes. He then took out the greens and began to eat them as matter-of-factly as someone eating spinach. He motioned to the pot for me to try some, but there was no way I would even consider trying them. After all, he could touch them without getting stung, and all I got when I tried was a lot of pain. After he finished the greens, he reheated the water, strained out the debris, sweetened it with some honey, and drank it like tea. No matter how much he tried to explain that the sting was taken away by the cooking and how good they tasted, he couldn't convince me to try it.

A few weeks later, Grandfather tricked me into eating nettle. He had collected some of the tender new top leaves from the plant, which looked nothing like the young shoots that he had collected weeks before. He cooked them up without my seeing and served them right along with the regular meal. I questioned him as to what type of green we were having, and he told me that it was a type of plantain. I had eaten plantain before so I ate the greens without hesitation, finding them very delicious. He laughed and told me what he had done, but I wouldn't believe him—that is, until he handed me a fresh leaf and it bit me. From then on, nettles and I have been good friends and one of my favorite wild foods.

Later on in the season, we learned what a fine cordage the fibers of nettle made. It still took some getting used to handling even the dried plant. I had a healthy respect for the sting and always gave it the benefit of the doubt. It wasn't until years later that I learned how to handle the plant without getting stung. I also learned that even though there is a knack to handling it with the hands, you will never learn to handle it with the body.

Food   Nettles are a very nourishing food, containing high levels of vitamins C and A, and also high levels of protein. New shoots and tiny pale green leaves can be boiled for fifteen minutes and eaten like spinach. The greens can also be boiled, then added to soups or stews. The water from the boiled greens can be strained, sweetened, and drunk like a tea, hot or cold. It will soon become one of your favorite wild edibles, but I do caution that the plant should be collected with gloves. It takes years and an intimate relationship with the plant before you can attempt to handle it without hand protection. Steaming the greens also works well. All species of nettle are edible.

Medicinal   A strong tea made from boiling the herb during the cooking is an aid to digestion and an appetite stimulant. It is also effective for urinary problems. Grandfather would use the nettle tea also as an external skin wash for minor infections and skin disorders. He would mix a strong tea with tallow and use it as a hand lotion for dried, chapped hands. I have found the tea to be effective in alleviating the bite of chiggers and mosquitoes, but there are better plants for this purpose. I strain the tea before drinking.

New Jersey Tea (*Ceanothus americanus*)

Description New Jersey tea is a lover of the dry, open woods. It is a low, bushy shrub, growing to about four inches tall. Its leaves are finely toothed with three prominent veins that curve toward the tip. Its flowers are in stalked, oval clusters originating from the upper leaf axils. The five-petaled flowers bloom from late spring right through the summer. The plants are found from Florida and Alabama, north into Canada.

Personality On any particularly long hikes to our outermost camp areas, we had a number of stops we would make along the way. These stops were not only to rest but also to replenish our water, eat, or gather materials needed for when we arrived at our outer camp. There was the spring stop on our way to the Wells Mills area, where we would get our water; there was the cattail stop, where we would collect some of our edibles; and there was the reed stop on the way to the old Cramer farm, where we would collect our arrow shafts. One stop in particular was always a favorite to us, and that was the tea stop on the way to our Jackson camp area.

The tea stop was located by a little spring, and the tea we used was the New Jersey tea plant. It was a ritual we had anytime we were headed to that particular area, and many times we would hike to the tea stop only to have the tea. We didn't always need the excuse of the Jackson campground to visit the spot. The tea had to be used dry so there was preparation involved each time we came to the area. The first thing we did was to make our tea, sit by the spring, and enjoy the whole effect just like the traditional Japanese tea ceremony. Before we left, we gathered and bound a handful of leaves for drying, placed them in a little bark dryer that we had built to store the leaves for future use, and headed on our way. The tea was easily one of my favorites.

The medicinal value of the tea did not surface until years after we were well acquainted with it. On one of Grandfather's visits to an old friend, we had the delight of taking part in the collecting and making of his friend's sinus remedy. Grandfather's friend Bill suffered from a chronic sinus condition that erupted every fall. Grandfather had shown Bill how to make a good sinus remedy out of the New Jersey tea root, and the procedure was undertaken every summer.

We dug up a few tea plants, bundled the leaves to dry, and collected the roots. The roots were washed and laid to dry on the rafters of the woodshed. A few weeks later we came back and helped Grandfather and Bill scrape the bark from the roots and store it in a small cotton bag. The sinus remedy was made by taking a small palmful of bark and steeping it in hot water for one-half hour. The tea was then taken twice a day during Bill's sinus season and seemed to work very well for him.

I had also gathered, dried, and prepared some rootbark for myself, feeling that I, too, might someday have sinus trouble, and stored it away in my medicine bag, virtually forgetting about it altogether. Months passed and we were in the mid-winter doldrums when I was hit with a cold. It was no ordinary cold, and I was quite congested and achy, and was suffering with a sinus headache. That's when I remembered the rootbark remedy Bill used, and I tried some on myself. To my dismay, the rootbark did not clear up my sinuses or get rid of the headache. The only thing that kept me from total disappointment was remembering Grandfather telling me that sometimes a remedy worked on one person but not another.

Later that afternoon, Rick stopped by my house to see how I was doing. I complained to him about my sinuses and how I had been disappointed over the results of the bark remedy. After discussing my cold, the remedy, and my inability to accompany him on the hike he was about to take, he said that I didn't seem that bad off. After all, I didn't even look like I had a cold. That's when I realized that I had, in fact, stopped sniffling, and my lung congestion and cough had cleared up. Despite the sinus headache, I wasn't feeling that bad either. The remedy had worked but not in the way I suspected.

I learned much from the bark remedy. I not only learned how a remedy or medication can affect each person differently, but my expectation had prejudiced my observation of the drug's overall effect on my cold. Grandfather was always telling us to have no expectations about anything. He said that if we had expectations we would be clouded with prejudice and anticipation that would block the enjoyment of things, possibly even filling us with undue disappointment because our expectations have not been met. Confucius' old saying, "To have no expectations is to have everything," really made sense from that day on.

Plants, I've learned, teach us far more than just how to heal ourselves or feed our bodies. Like all of nature, they can become dynamic teachers of philosophy, practicality, survival, and so much more. All we have to do is to open ourselves to the tiny voices and subtleties. Things beyond normal sight and sound can teach us a great deal. It seems that with every plant about which we learned, there was always so much more than just the physical lessons: There was a whole wealth of spiritual knowledge as well.

Food New Jersey tea is one of the finest teas there is. The new succulent leaves or the tiny top leaves make the best delicate teas. The older leaves make a more hearty brew. The leaves must be thoroughly dried and stored in a cotton bag or earthenware container. The tea is made by steeping a small palmful of crushed leaves in hot water for fifteen minutes, then strained and enjoyed like any herbal tea. Be careful not to drink in large quantities because of the medicinal values.

Medicinal Grandfather used to make an effective skin wash with New Jersey tea. He would collect the whole plant, the older the better, and steep it in hot water for forty-five minutes to one hour. The tea was then used as a skin wash for sores, abrasions, and skin maladies of all sorts. He also used it personally as a hair ointment before the final rinse. Adding the tea to tallow, he would also make an efficient balm for localized skin problems. It worked well on the few pimples I had when I was a teenager.

The dried bark of the root also makes a good medication. A palmful of the dried bark can be steeped in hot water for one-half hour and taken internally, two cups a day. It works as a sedative and an antihistamine. I use it as a remedy for the common cold or flu. It also makes a mouthwash and gargle, good for sore throats or tooth and gum pain. In addition, I find it also helps cold sores and sinus congestion.

Oak (*Quercus spp.*)

Description   These familiar trees, though having various leaf shapes and a variety of sizes, all contain the well-known acorn. The acorns are thin shelled and found nestled in a tiny basal cup. The acorn crops vary through the years and are depended upon heavily by all sorts of wildlife. Any time we collect from an oak, we should take into consideration the other forms of wildlife that need them also. I even go to the extent of planting some of the acorns to insure new trees in the future. The trees are very widespread, growing throughout the country in various soil conditions, many species with various ranges. The oaks are abundant from Minnesota to Maine and south throughout Oklahoma, to Texas and Georgia. They can also be found in New Mexico, but rarely northward into the northwest Pacific.

Personality   The Pine Barrens are primarily made up of pines and scrub oak. However, interspersed throughout the regions are areas made up of white and black oak, which grow quite large. Near one of our favorite swamps grew a huge white oak that we called Grandfather Oak. In its large upper branches, we lashed together a huge observation platform that afforded a spectacular view of the swamp. Animals were oblivious to our being around and went about their usual chores without fear. Over a period of years, we added on a small thatch hut, sand and rocks for a fire area, and an outer wall to further seclude us from the animals. It was a tree-top home as intricate as the one described in *The Swiss Family Robinson*. In fact, it was that story which inspired its construction.

We loved that old oak and were always careful never to damage any of its branches. We knew that tree as well as the squirrels did, forming our own little roadways along its branches that led to various smaller observation platforms found throughout the tree. To us it was a safe haven above the whole world. We visited it so often that the squirrels and raccoons who inhabited the area befriended us, showing no fear. It was always a holiday any time we camped on that platform. The adventures and the magic of the animal shows always filled our day.

During one of our fall campouts at the old oak, Grandfather came to visit. We had just finished lunch when Grandfather began to collect all the acorns that had fallen onto the platform. We instinctively began to help because we knew that we were about to learn something new about the oak. We then husked the acorns and diced up the soft nutty centers, placed them in a muslin bag, and put them into a fast-moving stream. Grandfather had us taste the acorn before placing it into the water so that we would know its bitter taste. He then left the camp for a few days and told us to leave the bag soaking in the stream.

A few days later he returned and retrieved the bag. When he had us taste the acorns again, we found them delicious with no trace of bitterness. We then lay them in the sun to dry, finally grinding them into a flourlike consistency, then drying the powder again. Taking water and a little foxtail-grass flour he mixed in the acorns and made them into ash cakes. These were absolutely delicious and very satisfying. It was strange, but we did not have to eat again until very late in the day. The one thing we knew about the oak flour was that it was highly nutritious and made a great survival food.

The same day, my usual case of poison ivy began to bother me very badly. Grandfather took a handful of acorn husks and boiled them for about an hour in a small pan of water. Once finished, he took the strong tea and wiped it onto my affected area, repeating the process every hour. By nightfall the itching had stopped and the swelling had subsided. He told us stories of using the tannic acid found in the acorns as one of the ancient hide tanning techniques, though it wasn't as nice a tan as that produced by brain tanning. We talked about the oak for hours discussing all its uses, our notebooks jammed full of information that would take a lifetime to assimilate.

The oak tree also taught us to make our first bows. It is a difficult wood to work and does not make the finest bow, but for survival situations, it is quite serviceable. We also used oak to make our baskets, backrests, tool handles, and many other things. Since oak is one of the strongest hardwoods in the Pine Barrens, and other hardwoods are in limited supply, we depended on our oak brother for many things. Even my first set of snowshoes and cross-country skis were made from oak saplings. Oak also made some of the best fire-hardened spears and fish arrows, a little heavy but very strong and durable. An oak is one of the best friends a survivalist can have, producing an abundance of food, medication, and practical uses.

Food One way to remove the bitter tannin from acorns is to boil the whole nuts in several changes of water. After the water no longer turns a reddish-brown, taste the acorn for bitterness. If it is still bitter, then boil again in a few more changes of water. One of my favorite things is to roast the nuts and eat them as you would almonds, or roll them in brown sugar to make a delicious nut candy.

Acorn flour is produced by grinding the nuts and is best mixed with another type of flour. It is highly nutritious, and high in protein and fats. Acorns can be substituted in any recipe calling for nuts.

During a cold winter campout, Grandfather produced a low-grade flour from the inner bark of an oak. He stripped away the inner bark and boiled it in several changes of water, then air-dried it until it was nearly brittle. He then ground this into a serviceable flour, but it was not quite as good as the flour made from the acorns. At other times, during dire survival situations when food was scarce, we would cook the tiny oak rootlets in several changes of water, then add them to stews or salads. It was important to gather only the tiniest rootlets, for the older ones become much too bitter and stringy.

Medicinal Oak has a high concentration of tannic acid, especially in its acorns. I always make a point of saving the first boiling of the acorn preparation for use later on as an astringent skin wash. This skin wash is good for all skin irritations, pimples, boils, bee stings, poison ivy, and many other things. A stronger tea can be brewed from the acorn husks and is used for bad cases of poison ivy, and even fungal infections. I find that the tea also makes a good gargle for sore throats, gum problems, and is especially effective on cold sores.

A mild tea from the second or third boiling of the acorn preparation is good for many internal problems. It is an effective enema for hemorrhoids and also can be taken internally to reduce fever or stop internal bleeding. The tea for internal use should be made by boiling a small palmful of dried bark in one cup of water for twenty minutes. No more than two cups a day should be taken and not for more than two days. The bitter liquid can be sweetened with honey to make it more palatable. I find that it also makes a good tea for aiding digestion or as a tonic during the cold season. Stronger teas are made from the red-oak group and milder teas from the white-oak group, depending on the dosage, patient, illness, and condition.

Pine (*Pinus spp.*)

Description   Pine is a very familiar evergreen of all shapes, sizes, and locations. It is a cone-bearing tree with slender needles along the twigs. Needles are bound at base in bundles from two to five, depending on the species of pine. Whereas female cones are large and woody, male cones are soft, fleshy, and produce pollen. One or more species are common to all parts of the country in most soils. Individual species may vary.

Personality   There is a very special place in my heart for pines, especially the pitch pine. Pines have always been part of my life and are the first real trees I ever saw. I grew up in the Pine Barrens; the trees were my teachers, and the forests my home. Pines have fed me in times of famine and cared for me in sickness. They have given me shelter when there was none other about, and they make any survival situation easier. The pitch pine, which is the dominant pine of the forests where I grew up, is not a very pretty pine at first glance. It does not meet the textbook type of requirements we think of when we think pine. It is short—never over thirty feet—and is sparsely branched, bent, gnarled, and otherwise misshapen and unsymmetrical. Once you begin to know these pines, you are forever hooked on their artistic beauty and their individuality, and mystified by the way they grow in the harshest of conditions.

The Pine Barrens of New Jersey were my proving grounds, my classroom, and my anvil. They forged my beliefs, sharpened my skills, and introduced me to the world of nature. They were an unyielding teacher. It was so easy to get lost, for there were no real ridges or landmarks; all trees were nearly the same height, and the underbrush of scrub oak, brier, and blueberry was at times nearly impenetrable. The Pinelands did not give up their secrets easily, for the animals could effortlessly conceal themselves, as the sandy forest floor did not give to tracks easily. By far, especially during the winter months, they made survival near impossible. They yielded little, yet taught so much.

It stands to reason that the first plant I ever learned about was the pine. Sure I knew its name long before I knew there was a Stalking Wolf, but Grandfather gave me my first introduction to what now has become a very intimate relationship. I know that no matter where there is a pine, my survival is insured. It was the pine forests that fueled my lust for survival, tracking, and adventure, but it was also the pine itself that caused me to fall in love with plants. It was that first introduction into the world of the plant people that has kept me obsessed with plants all these years, and it shows no signs of letting up. The pine has become my gateway, my symbol, to the deeper world of plants.

It wasn't long after I met Grandfather that I was introduced to my pine brothers and sisters. To Rick and me, Grandfather was the spirit of the wilderness. He seemed to contain all the knowledge we ever wanted to know, and through his stories he uplifted our spirits, put wilderness adventure into our imaginations, and brought us closer to the Earth in a very loving way. For weeks on end we sat listening to his wisdom. He could tell us new things about the landscape we never realized, show us animals that we would have otherwise passed, and make us feel that the Earth was alive. He spoke of kinship in all life and that we could reach a oneness where we would no longer be alien to the natural world. Once we reached that oneness we could survive anywhere with our bare hands as our only resources.

The adventure of survival without depending on manufactured things intrigued us more than anything else. We had just gotten into camping and our packs and equipment were cumbersome, very much like a chain that held us to one place. It seemed that, in order to go into the woods, we had to carry a lifeline from civilization, a permanently attached umbilical cord to the security of the artificial. That cord destroyed our freedom and restricted our movement. We would never really be free and wild as long as we had to depend on all those things to keep us alive. We would never truly know a oneness with all things. At best, all we could be was a small part of the overall picture.

Grandfather started us off slowly. At first he taught us to build a debris hut that looked like a rather large but snug squirrel nest. The debris hut weaned us from the sleeping bag and tent, and the bow drill made it possible to have fire anyplace. After six months of pretend camping and sleeping in the back yard, we were ready for our first test. It was the first time we were to camp out in the woods without the aid of sleeping bags or matches. We carried with us the usual umbrella tent and sleeping bag to keep our parents happy, but quickly discarded these when we were out of sight of the house. We made camp easily and got a fire going, feeling quite competent in taking care of the first three necessities: shelter, water, and fire.

It was on this campout that we were first introduced to pine in a real way. Sure, we knew the tree as a thing of interest, a place to climb, or a place of shade, but Grandfather changed our opinion of the pine, and subsequently altered our awareness of plants in general. From that point in time on, we never looked at plants or any other entity of nature in the same way again. When the work of camp was done, we all sat down to relax. Rick and I planned the areas we would explore, and Grandfather boiled some water. He eventually asked us if we would like some tea, and we, of course, agreed whole-heartedly, hoping that it would be one of the special brews that he carried with him.

Instead of reaching into his bag for the tea as he had done in the past, he walked slowly over to a small head-high pine. We watched him as he inspected the tree, finally pulling off what amounted to a handful of newer needles forming a few boughs. Back at camp, he began to dice up the needles, producing a handful of tiny little pieces. He dumped these into hot water and took the pot off the fire. We didn't say a word, watching the whole procedure carefully. Part of me could not believe that he was making a tea from pine. I was fascinated, almost spellbound. For the first time I was witnessing something we had only heard stories about—living off the wild plants.

At the end of a period of time that seemed an eternity, Grand-father poured us a cup of tea. I expected it to taste as it smelled: bitter, piny, and full of resin. What I drank was an absolutely delicious cup of tea. It was like none I had ever tasted before. Its wild but mild taste seemed to bind us to the forest and to the tree itself. There, drinking that tea, we had a small hint of what it was like to have a part of the natural world become part of our lives. We felt intimately connected to that little pine, and through the years we watched it grow. To us it was truly a brother and now it stands over twenty feet tall, strong and straight, probably due to the way we constantly fussed over it throughout all these years. Every time I pass that tree with one of my classes, it reminds me of the first taste of the wild. Unfor-tunately, the area is slated for development.

On our next campout, we learned more about pine. We were learning how to make arrow shafts and were nearly finished attaching the feathers. Grandfather pulled us away from our work temporarily, and we went gathering pine pitch. We scraped the pitch from old wounds. Hard or soft, it was all taken. He compared the pitch to blood, and taught us to leave a good coating of resin on the tree to prevent infection. Back at camp, we heated the pitch until it was a thick gooey mess, filled with bits of debris, and dark brown in color. We strained the mess through a grass filter and repeated the process until all foreign matter was removed.

The pitch now resembled amber-colored model glue. We heated it up once again and collected the fine white wood ash from our fire. Grandfather picked up a little pitch on the end of a clean stick, lightly coated the arrow wrappings, then dusted the ash into place. This turned the resin gray-black and hardened it tremendously. It wasn't like the sticky or gooey globs that were found on fresh tree wounds that never seem to harden. This resin was hard enough to sand down smooth, but not so hard as to be brittle. It was sort of an ancient epoxy-resin. The resins of pine have been used to fill cracks in pots, to join wood, to waterproof wrappings, to attach fish hooks firmly, and for hundreds of other jobs. It truly amazed us that we never seemed to run out of uses of the pine.

Food   One of the first times we put pine to a test as a real survival food was during a winter campout. We had built camp on a Friday evening but did not have a chance to hunt or gather anything to eat. We woke the next morning to nearly a foot of snow, accompanied by high winds and bitterly cold temperatures. We took a few hours to build a fire and make an awning on our shelter to keep the wind and blowing snow away, but that was not enough. We were growing very hungry and trips out were limited to only a few minutes at a time. That's when Grandfather showed us how to make flour from the inner bark of pine.

We located a pine near camp that had been cut down by the forest fire service. It had only been cut a few days before and was relatively fresh, despite the fact that it was dying. We cut the rest of the stump away, cleaned off the limbs, and dragged it back to camp. Here we scraped off the outer bark and stripped off long sheaths of inner bark. Grandfather dried these on a makeshift rack next to the fire until they were hard and a bit brittle. We ground up the dry inner bark to a flourlike consistency and made it into ash cakes. These ash cakes were delicious and very substantial, even though they were a little resiny tasting. Grandfather said that in an emergency we could remove the bark from live trees without killing the tree. We could peel away long horizontal strips to get our inner bark, provided that once we were better off we would come back and paint the tree with hot pitch to protect the wound.

We also learned that the pollen from the male cones is very edible. It is great mixed with flour, used as a stew thickener, or sprinkled atop any grain cereal. The firm young male cones of pine can be boiled and used also as an emergency survival food. The diced needles, young or old, can be used to make a tea that is rich in vitamins A and C. Ripe pine cones can be opened by placing them next to a fire. The seeds can be roasted and eaten or ground into a high-grade flour. In times of need I have even cooked and eaten the rootlets of pine, preparing them like a potherb by boiling them in two changes of water for twenty-five minutes.

Medicinal   One of the best uses of pine I know of, and have used with great success, is as a bandage. I use the fresh supple inner bark and tie it onto the wound much the same way I would use a swath of clean cotton cloth. If the wound is bad, I will use fresh, clean sphagnum moss as the dressing, held into place by the inner bark. Sphagnum moss has been used for years as bandages, diapers, and poultices for wounds of all types. I find that a poultice of inner bark is also a good drawing salve for insect bites or boils. It is best not to let the inner bark dry out when used as a bandage.

Plantain (*Plantago major*)

Description   Plantain is a lover of lawns, gardens, roadsides, and fields. Leaves of the common plantain are in basal rosettes, found low to the ground. The greenish-white and tiny flowers are found along leafless stems. The leaves are roundish, heavily ribbed, and very broad with flattened stems. It flowers from summer to mid-fall. One or more species of plantain is found throughout the United States.

Personality   Grandfather was born in 1874 on the border of what is now New Mexico and Texas. After his father, mother, and grandfather were killed in a land skirmish, he moved with his great-grandfather to northeast Mexico in the hot mountainous, desert regions known today as the Chiricahua Mountain Range. He was barely two years old at the time, and was raised for the next twenty-one years under the tutelage of his great-grandfather. Most of the people in that little village were quite old, and Stalking Wolf was being groomed to understand the old ways. Because of the traditional life-style and beliefs of the old ones, no white-man possessions were permitted in camp, so his education was of the old ways. He grew to be the scout, warrior, and, eventually, medicine man of his little group. Most of the younger people that he knew were being moved to reservations in the United States, and for all purposes, he and his people were fugitives.

They were left quite alone since the land was of little use to the white man or Mexicans. Most of the area was harsh, hot, and barren, creating a natural barrier between his people and the wars going on in the outside world. He learned his lessons well, proving himself a powerful hunter, protector, and warrior. His fame spread rapidly among the surrounding Apache groups. Grandfather was a loner, sometimes traveling hundreds of miles in search of game or to scout out potential enemy threats. He was a master of stalking, camouflage, and evasion, for his life depended on his cunning and his ability to escape detection. He could travel for many months and miles in all types of weather carrying with him just a small bag of seeds, a bone knife, and a loin cloth. He had to make all the things he needed for survival since he could not carry much with him.

During his regular training in scouting, tracking, survival, nature awareness, and all the other necessary physical skills, he was also being trained in the world of the spiritual. The gateway to the spiritual world was through the medicinal plants and how they could be used to heal. His great-grandfather was also a coyote teacher who

169

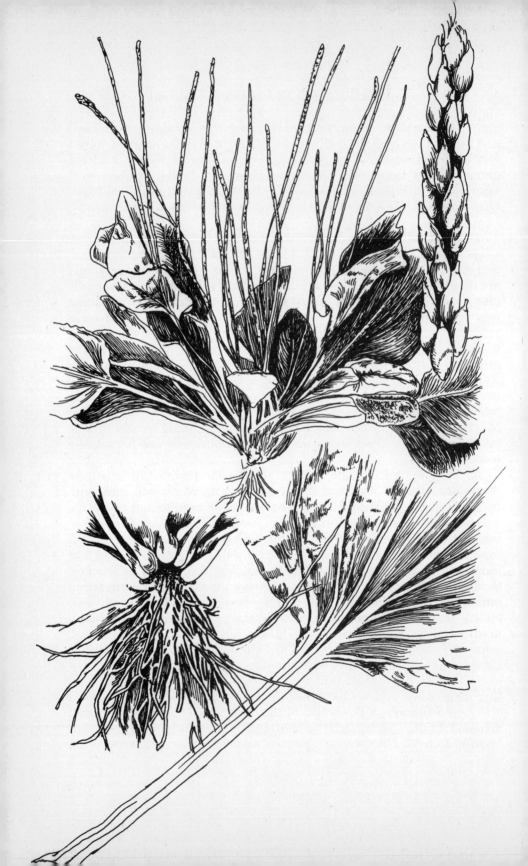

had Stalking Wolf discover things for himself, thus building his own beliefs and personal medicine. The Visionary Experience was also important to Grandfather, and he frequently visited the mountains alone for periods of fasting, prayer, and vision seeking. This all led to his questioning of some of the old ways and customs, which started him on his quest to learn new things.

He was a wanderer. Leaving his people just after his great-grandfather died, he wandered all over this country. His travels took him as far south as Panama and as far north as Alaska. Most of the time was spent wandering this country, visiting the elders, then incorporating their teachings into his belief system. His thirst for knowledge and spiritual enlightenment took him far and wide. I never realized how much he knew until years after he departed. The skills that he passed down to us were the absolute best of many tribes, not just Apache. They covered a wide variety of situations and techniques, always suited to fit the area, borrowed from so many cultures. Grandfather, then, was not strictly Apache, nor did he follow the Apache faith all the way. He was a child of the universe that encouraged us to drop off the old ways that did not prove out in nature and follow our own path.

He was very Emersonian in approach. Each man was his teacher and he listened to everyone. Nature became his proving ground, his university, and the holiest of temples. He cared little where he learned a valuable skill, whether it came from whites, blacks, yellows, or reds, for he believed that we were all children of the Earth. He taught us bows of Apache and Mohawk design, nets from the Quinault, and fishing techniques of the Penobscot. He also showed us many things introduced to him by the white man. Most Apaches had a great fear and respect for water and would not go into anywhere they could not see the bottom. Grandfather learned from the Penobscots not to fear the water and thus loved any body of water. After I wrote *The Tracker*, letters began to pour in from all over the country, telling stories of meeting Grandfather many years before in his travels.

This little bit of history thus brings me to the plantain. Many traditional Native Americans would not eat plantain because it was brought here by the white man. The plant grew in the white man's fields and grasslands and was considered by many a form of bad medicine because of this close association. Grandfather cared little for that kind of superstition. He realized how the plant got here, and in his mind it was still owned by the Creator and was thus sacred. The knowledge of the plant's edibility also came to him when he was traveling in upper New York. An old white hermit took him in for a few days and passed along much of his folklore. One plant he learned about was the plantain.

At first, Grandfather was very skeptical and fearful about using the plant. He still somewhat clung to the old traditions. After a plantain poultice took the sting out of a bee sting and immediately deadened the pain and swelling, Grandfather adopted the plant. From that day on, no matter a man's color, religion, or overall beliefs, Grandfather listened and learned, dropping away his own prejudices. I doubt very much if Grandfather would have known half of what he did when he was with us if he had stuck only to one way of life and one tradition. Everything interested him and he made sure that we were taught to drop away prejudice and open ourselves to the truth, no matter where it originates or who teaches us.

Food   One of our neighbors was out weeding his garden when Grandfather and I passed by on our way to the swimming hole. Next to him was a huge pile of what he considered to be worthless weeds. Grandfather politely asked him if he could take some of the weeds because they would make a good meal. Looking a little shocked, the man easily agreed, glad to get rid of the useless things. We stuffed the pile into a makeshift bag made from a blanket and headed off to the water's edge. We spread the greens down on the blanket and found that most of them consisted of plantain. Grandfather and I spent a little time collecting the newest baby leaves until the pile was exhausted and we had quite a few.

We discarded the larger leaves into Grandfather's tobacco patch for mulch, then went swimming and exploring for a few hours. We got back to the camp utterly famished. Grandfather lit a fire and began to boil some water, putting in the plantain greens, then simmering them for a little over fifteen minutes. The result was an absolutely delicious spinachlike meal. Its taste was far different than the garden spinach, richer and more wild tasting. I could tell the effect it had on my body, how it had far more food value than the usual garden spinach. The next morning we nibbled on the remainder of the raw leaves before returning to my house. Since then, I have been chopping up the leaves and making them a standard addition to all of my salads, wild or otherwise.

All the way back to the house, Grandfather and I were in deep discussion as to why people refer to plants as weeds or junk wood. To me, they were alien terms, because every plant I knew had some use or another. Some of them were very critical to survival conditions and I could not have made it through many an outing without them. Grandfather said that most people's feet are removed from the soil and the wisdom of their ancient ancestors. Because of cultivated crops and other customs, many plants and animals have little or no use to modern man, which is why he is so apt to destroy them without a second thought.

Plants are either edible, medicinal, or utilitarian in some way. Grandfather stated emphatically that even if we did not know the use of a plant, we should consider its importance to the overall plan of the natural world. Nothing has been put on this Earth without a very definite purpose. I interrupted him and asked about poison ivy. He told me, rather angrily but still understanding, that poison ivy was one of the most powerful catalysts and medications we have. Without poison ivy, certain remedies of his would not work. It is also food for many animals during the lean months of the season. Birds will eat the seeds, and the smaller rodents and rabbits eat the end buds. To remove poison ivy could kill many animals and take away many of our important medications. Nothing is without a powerful purpose, whether man understands or not.

I parch the seeds of the common plantain, dry and winnow them and add them to salads or breads. I also grind them into a low-grade flour and mix them with other flours to produce a fine bread, or I nibble them after roasting. I make a peanut-butter substitute by mixing partially dried and crushed seeds with equal parts butter. I find it much better than peanut butter and prefer it most of the time. I also make cookies using a peanut-butter-cooky recipe, only substituting with the plantain butter.

Medicinal   One of the first medicinal uses of plantain I witnessed was with one of Grandfather's patients. This person had a very badly infected wound which oozed pus and bled periodically. All the store-bought things the man tried only increased the pain and did little to heal the wound. Out of desperation, the man called on Grandfather, even though he did not fully believe in herbalists or herbal remedies. Grandfather made a poultice from plantain leaves that he had gathered, telling us that it made little difference whether it was common or seaside plantain. He applied the poultice to the wound.

The next day when the dressing and the poultice were removed, the swelling and discharge of pus were nonexistent. The gentleman commented that after Grandfather had left, the pain had all but subsided. Grandfather then made a strong tea of plantain leaves steeped in hot water for thirty minutes. This warm tea was wiped onto the infected area. The patient was to repeat the process twice a day for the next two days. The next time we saw the man, the wound was completely healed and had no scarring. The man became a believer in herbology despite the fact that he was a retired doctor.

The strong tea made by taking a palmful of plantain leaves and steeping in warm water for forty-five minutes is good for many other ailments. It makes a good mouthwash for cold sores and gum problems, and I have found it effective in treating toothaches. It also makes a good skin wash for most skin maladies and has an ability to slow down blood flow from a mild cut. Most of all, a mild tea of the leaves makes a good cough remedy and is great for breaking up congestion. I also use it as a vitamin substitute, eating a few green seeds every day. It seems to act as an internal insecticide, possibly rendering the skin tasteless to insects.

Reed (*Phragmites communis*)

Description   The reed is a tall, stately plant, jointed, hollow or pithy. Its leaves are long and elegant, topped with a silky, plumelike flower cluster, which is purplish when young, but turns whitish-gray when older. The leaves are gray-green in appearance, and the rootstock is very long, forming a thick mat in mud. It is a lover of fresh or brackish marshes, ditches, and damp roadsides. Reed is found from Maine, south to Maryland, Ohio, and Illinois, and also in Louisiana, Texas, and Mexico.

Personality   I stand at the edge of what once was a huge sand dune and look out over Barnegat Bay. It is mid-winter, cold and windy, and as far as the eye can see there are reed jungles. They ebb and flow with the wind like some golden-brown sea, casting waves here and there, trembling at times, as they await the next gust or ripple in concentric rings. At first glance, they appear as one unit, as consistent as water; yet at other times, they are as individual as people, each with its separate personality. Here, twenty-five years after I discovered them, my mind slips into periods of reverie, drifting back to the times we first played in these jungles and how fascinated we were with them.

My first trip to the reed jungles was to gather reeds for arrow shafts. Despite their flimsy appearance, they make the fastest arrow shafts I have ever known. Their speed makes it possible to drive an arrow clear through a deer, unless they hit a bone. For smaller and faster game, they were the absolute best. We spent hours that first day, collecting and drying the shafts that were still faintly green with summer's energy. They were unlike any plant we had previously encountered. Even the close cattail bore only a slight resemblance. The most fascinating thing about reeds was the way they worked in unison with each other and the wind. Only the smaller grasses exhibited this tendency but none were as choreographed as the reed.

Reed patches were always a special place full of wonders and adventures. We could become lost and disoriented in them for hours. The magic of discovery never seemed to end. Marsh hawks drifted above, muskrats on the waters, birds and beasts of all description throughout. If we were to spend more than a few hours in the reeds we would soon make our own pathways that integrated with those the animals had created. They would blend into a beautiful sequence of roadways that we became very familiar with. We would practice stalking, camouflage, and playing a form of hide-and-seek to sharpen our skills.

When the prospects of camping in the reed jungles finally came up, we were eager to go. It was one of the last weeks of summer and a welcome last campout before the prison of school took away our seemingly endless freedom. We built our shelter by pulling huge sections of the reeds together so they formed a low dome. Then we burrowed into them. Stacking more dead leaves on top, we had homes much like muskrat domes when viewed at a distance. Even in the rain we stayed snug and warm. The tubelike insulation of the plants helped hold our heat. Within the eternity of the day, we built ourselves a minicommunity, connected to and part of the reed world, so we felt as one with it. Even the smaller animals and birds shared our shelters. Their voices and rustling produced beautiful night music.

The next day we found Grandfather by the bay's edge. He had collected five huge bundles of reed, which he had then bounded together to resemble a log raft. Pulling together the ends of this raft and binding them into a blunt point, he had created what looked like a fat canoe. To this he added an outrigger of another reed bundle, fastened to the main boat with stout staffs. He pulled himself out of the canals and into the coves where he went around the end point, returning in a few moments. We expected him to be wet with the water that would soak through the floor but he came out totally dry. The boat was very light, buoyant, and very maneuverable.

By mid-afternoon, Rick and I had built ourselves reed boats, too. Though not as sophisticated as Grandfather's, they worked quite well. We spent the remainder of the day in our boats, exploring the outer fringes of the reed jungles. The next day we used our boats to cross the bay to do some clamming and to explore the outer mud flats. Remarkably, these boats lasted the entire fall and we used them again the next spring and part of the summer. By that time we had learned to make reed mats, thatch huts, baskets, fish traps, and spears. The reed offered us never-ending possibilities of survival tools. All we had to do was use our imagination.

The first use of the reed as a food came to us that same campout. Grandfather had us keep near camp all the tops of the reeds. We spent hours shaking the seedheads onto a buckskin mat, collecting a huge pile of the tiny reddish seeds. These we parched, winnowed, and ground into a coarse flour. We mixed the flour with wild blackberries and made tasty ash cakes. The next morning, we cooked the unground seeds into a type of porridge that tasted absolutely delicious. I prefer reed porridge to that of oatmeal. At other times during the campout, we added reed flour to our stews and soups or used it as breading on our fish.

There is a certain inexplicable tranquillity found within the confines of the reed jungles. In the fall, when the insects are but a distant memory, I find great peace sitting within their seclusion. The movement has the same tranquilizing effect on the human soul as does water, and their swaying with the wind is as hypnotizing as a pendulum. You can lie back and listen to the ancient and wild call of the waterfowl, listen to the scurry of mice, or the continuous symphony of birds. The reed jungles are as individual as the area in which they are found. Each jungle produces its own music and movement, some fast and abrupt, others slow and soothing, always in harmony with the animals that inhabit them, always a haven.

Food   One of our favorite foods came from the reed and was always a treat. We called it "bay candy" and were always eager in the spring to make some. We collected the fleshy green reed shoots, and then dried them in the sun. These we pounded into a stringy powder and dried them some more. We would add water to this fine powder and place on bark slabs, then slowly roast them next to a fire. This took on the consistency and look of roasted marshmallow and tasted just as good, if not better. The fresh fall or early spring roots of the reed can be collected and made into a fine flour, using the same method as for cattail root.

Medicinal   The medicinal uses of the reed are few. Most of the uses as a medicine are found in its catalytic properties. I find that the flour from the fresh root made into a paste or a poultice is a great relief for insect bites, especially those of mosquitoes. I usually use it for those bites that are persistent and swollen. I place the poultice or dough on the bite, then tie it on with a braid of reed leaves. I remove it after it dries.

I know a few old-timers that use a little of the old seed heads as an additive to tobacco. It tends to make the tobacco very strong and a little bitter tasting. I use the old flowerheads as a scrub pad when cleaning areas of irritated skin, especially poison ivy rash. It seems to be a combination of the brackish water and the scrub action of the flowerheads that temporarily relieve the itch.

Rose (*Rosa spp.*)

Description   Roses form a wide and extensive group of easily recognizable plants. They are bristly or thorny shrubs bearing beautiful five-petaled flowers that can be either pink or red. The fruit of the rose is bright red and appears in late summer and early fall, sometimes lasting throughout the winter. They are found in dry open woods, field edges, sandy areas, and in a variety of other terrains throughout the United States.

Personality   To me, rosebushes are the protectors of the small animal life. In any huge tangle of roses you will be sure to find a myriad of tunnels, trails, runs, hides, and bedding areas as well as an assortment of other animal signs. The rose tangles remind me of huge cities where high concentrations of animals live and work. They are every bit as impenetrable as brier patches and just as painful for those who don't take care going into them. They are by far the thickest of all protective areas and usually house the largest assortment of animals. To Rick and me, they were always a source of absorbing study, for at any time, we could see countless animals.

The wild rosebush patches found in the Pine Barrens were few and far between. They were usually located on the edges of old abandoned farm fields near some deserted town or homestead. The fields produced the food for all the herbivores of the area, and the bushes provided a most impenetrable protection. So many times, we saw foxes stop dead in their tracks at the edge of the rose tangles as their perspective prey vanished down the complicated maze of tunnels. Owls and hawks almost never ventured into them; any that did usually had to spend a long time pulling the dislodged rose thorns from their flesh. Only the weasels would venture down these tunnels but even then, they could not get to the bird population that nested in the upper strata without getting their feet full of thorns.

We found that if we carefully pulled ourselves into the rose patches, we would be able to watch the lives of animals unfold before us, unhindered by our presence. For some reason, the animals felt safe in these rose jungles and paid almost no attention to us. Many of them would walk within inches of our faces and, in a few cases, crawl right over our backs if we were obstructing one of their well-traveled trails. One of our favorite times was during the late spring when the flowers were in bloom. Not only could we witness the movement of animals and their songs, but our senses would become intoxicated by the rich fragrances that surrounded us. It was a most sensual experience.

To add even more dimension to our overloaded senses as we lay in the rose tunnels, we would feast on the rose petals. It tended to round out the experience so that all our senses would be involved in the action. This made us feel very close to the rose patches and a part of the natural world protected beneath its rough exterior. It was a secure haven from the outside world, full of adventures and new discoveries. In winter, unlike other brush tangles, the bare stems and shoots were just as impenetrable and protecting. Many of the animals that would inhabit the other brush tangles of the area in the summer would migrate to the rose tangles in winter. The population beneath the roses would increase substantially and give us much more to look at. We would dine on rose hips as a replacement for the rose petals. These were out of the weather and protected still in the bosom of the roses.

One of our late fall duties was to collect the rose hips to make winter tonic to help prevent colds and other illnesses. We would collect the berries, taking care to leave plenty for the animals. We would then remove the seeds and dry the fleshy hips in the warm fall sun, then grind up the dried hips into a coarse powder and dry again to insure thorough dryness. To this we would add equal parts rose petals that we had collected and dried in the spring. This would become our stash. Grandfather would have us drink a half cup of rose tea throughout the flu-infested winter months to help us stay healthy. It worked well as we were rarely sick even with common colds, although half of our school would be out sick. The one winter I failed to use the tonic, I had more colds and flu than I had in my whole life previously.

Food Not only were the rose patches a source of intense animal study, but they also provided us with food, medication, and many practical uses in a survival situation. The fresh rose petals are excellent as a trailside nibble, added to salads, or made into teas. These are delicious, having a taste unique to them. If you love tea, you will love mixing your favorite tea with dried or fresh rose petals. The smell of the tea becomes almost intoxicating and will give you a new taste sensation. The fleshy part of the rose hip can be eaten raw or dried and made into tea the same way as petal tea. Rose hips are very high in vitamin C and that could be one of the reasons that they make an excellent winter tonic. Rose hips make an excellent emergency survival food because they usually remain on the bush throughout the winter.

Medicinal   Strong rose tea made from the fresh or dried petals and hips makes a great skin wash for infections and inflammations. Strong doses of tea can also be effectively used as a mouthwash for many oral maladies. It also has a sedative effect which I commonly use for headaches or upset stomach. It is best to collect the rose petals before they bloom, as that is when they provide the most medicinal value. I have also used the warm tea as ear drops, allowing it to trickle into the infected ear.

Stronger medications can be made by mixing petals and hips with hot wine. A small palmful of petals and hips added to a cup of wine is the usual dosage. Use one-quarter cup twice a day internally or as an astringent for the skin. One favorite concoction that Grandfather used to make for the onset of colds was a mixture of yarrow and rose hips. This he brewed into a strong tea and drank two cups a day. He also used it on a few patients to help induce sweating, break fevers, and fortify the body against attacking germs.

Sassafras (*Sassafras albidum*)

Description   Sassafras is a medium-sized tree with leaves that can be ovate, or have two or three lobes. The edges are smooth with branched green twigs, whereas the older bark is reddish-brown. Leaves and twigs are very aromatic when scraped or crushed. The fruit is found on a reddish stalk with fleshy blue fruit containing one seed. It is a lover of transition areas and old fields. Its fruit can be found in the fall. Sassafras is found from Maine, west to Michigan, and south to Arkansas, Tennessee, and Virginia.

Personality   Rick and I loved to read. Our favorite books were always field guides or animal stories, but a close second were adventure stories and novels. One summer we were both reading *Tom Sawyer*, taking turns reading to each other in the campfire light. We were especially taken by the part where Tom took a trip down the Mississippi River on a raft he and Huck Finn had built. Since both our houses were located on the Toms River and since we always wanted to explore it by boat, we made plans to build a raft. We would build the raft upstream in a place we called Turtle Run and float the eight miles of river to our houses, stopping frequently to camp. We had plans for how we would build the fire platform, the rudder, the box house, and even the poles and makeshift sails. The only hitch was that we would not cut trees for such an adventure. That kind of senselessness was beyond our comprehension, and even the lure of future exciting adventures would not break down our convictions.

While hiking up to the Turtle Run area, we smelled the rich aroma of fresh-cut wood, accompanied by the roar of a chain saw. We knew that someone was clearing another woodlot to build a house, so we went to investigate. Finding the area and a good pile of straight logs that would be suitable for a raft, we asked the woodcutter if we could have them. Since there were very few woodstoves in use in that part of town, he willingly parted with the logs calling them junk trees. We asked him what type of wood it was, and he told us that it was sassafras. He added that it was junk wood because it wasn't good for anything and usually burned too fast for a wood stove.

We gratefully took the logs, which were not junk wood to us. In fact, we considered nothing in nature junk or a weed. The one thing we instantly noticed about the trees as we dragged them down to the river's edge was their very deep, intoxicating aroma that tended to make the mouth water. As we cut the logs and lay them together, we were constantly bathed in the rich fragrance, until our clothes,

181

hands, and body became saturated with the scent. Even my mother commented on the scent I had on my clothing that night at dinner. My brother sneered and said that it was a welcome change.

We spent quite a few days putting together our little raft. Though it looked like a log jam and was made of the so-called junk wood, it was very sturdy and floated well. On the appointed day of our launch of the week-long trip, we were surprised that Grandfather wanted to join us. He was as like a little kid, as excited and full of adventurous expectation as we were. We climbed aboard and slowly drifted the first few miles down the junglelike river. The day was absolutely beautiful, sunny, still, with turtles sunning on logs, birds all about adding their beautiful voices to the harmony of the frogs and buzz of insects. I took the rudder, Rick caught fish, and Grandfather relaxed as he eagerly surveyed the riverscape.

We edged the raft into a thick marshy area to spend the night. Rick cleaned the fish, I broke up pieces of firewood, and Grandfather pulled up some cattail to eat with the fish. We were just about to start the fire when we found that we had forgotten to pack the bow drills. There was no way we could wade to shore and get some wood for a bow drill because of the mud that would easily swallow a boy. Without saying a word, Grandfather took a piece of our sassafras cabin and began to carve a bow drill. Within fifteen minutes we had a roaring fire going and the meal cooking. As we waited, we told Grandfather the story of the woodcutter and how he had called the sassafras a junk wood. All of us had a good laugh because Grandfather explained to us that sassafras was not only one of the best bow-drill woods but also provided us with food, medicine, and had many other useful attributes.

As the days passed, we seemed to live effortlessly on the bounties of the river world. It was a magical place, one we had never really known until we gained our new perspective. The currents carried us by many unsuspecting animals. Being nearly invisible, we learned much about their secret lives. Our stops would bring us to small islands and groves of trees we could never have reached from the land routes. We stopped frequently at any provocation just to savor the unlimited amount of delights. It was during one of these impromptu stops that we were introduced further to our brother sassafras.

Grandfather steered us to a small tree that grew on a sandy point of land. Here was a little sassafras, and we would learn of its goodness. We studied it carefully, scraped a small twig, and out came the familiar fragrance. He carefully selected a handful of twigs and a large root from one of the smaller plants. He was meticulous in this removal, for he wanted to insure that the plant would not be hurt. He took the twigs and broke them up, putting them into hot water to steep. He then washed the root, diced some up, and added it to the hot water. The rest of the root was left to dry atop the shelter. He kept the water hot but not boiling for a little over a half hour until the liquid turned a deep reddish-brown. The tea was soothing and delicious. It seemed to take the chill out of the cool night and warm us to the core. Sassafras has since become one of my favorite teas.

Food   The root of the sassafras tree can be used fresh or dried. To dry the root, clean thoroughly, slice lengthwise, and allow it to dry in the warm sun. Chop the fresh or dried roots up into tiny chunks and add a palmful to two cups of hot water. While keeping the water warm, steep for about a half hour until the water turns a reddish-brown. Longer steeping time produces stronger teas. The roots can be used several times before they run out of flavor. Drink the tea just as you would regular tea, and sweeten to taste.

The young and succulent leaves can be dried, rubbed between the palms into a powder, and used as a stew thickener. It also makes a good flavoring for breads, breading for fish, and even as a standby tea stash. It is important to dry these leaves slowly in a gentle sun so as not to drive off too much of the flavor.

Warning: *Sassafras tea has been found to cause cancer in laboratory animals.* In my estimation, it would take the drinking of twelve cups a day for the rest of your life to get the proper dosage to cause any cancer. Remember, moderation in all things.

Medicinal   My first medicinal experience with sassafras was brought to me by an old piny chap named Jake. He was an old clammer who lived not far from the town of Barnegat, and I visited him frequently, learning from him how to clam, make crab traps, and how to go eeling with spears. We had known each other for quite a few years, and like all old people, he was a virtual storehouse of knowledge. Jake drank sassafras tea every day as a tonic to ward off illness. Listening to him speak of sassafras, I could feel his awe and respect for the plant.

I had gotten a bad skin infection from a cut I received while collecting cordage plants to make the nets. For a number of days it had grown more and more infected until it was very swollen and painful. I really believed that I was well on the way to blood poisoning and that I would have to cut my trip short. Jake examined my cut, brewed up some very strong sassafras tea from the root bark of the plant, then applied it to my wound. The first thing I noticed was that the pain almost disappeared, the redness disappeared soon after, and the swelling was completely down a few hours later. It healed quickly from that point on.

Sassafras has many more uses. The bark of the tree itself makes a mild medication while the bark of the root is much stronger. Either of them can be used as a mouthwash and both are good medications for killing pain, inducing sweating, and relieving rheumatism. They also have an ability to bring down a fever. I once again must stress that extracts of sassafras tea have been shown to cause cancer.

Shepherd's Purse (*Capsella bursa-pastoris*)

Description   Shepherd's purse is a lover of waste grounds, roadsides, and old fields. It bears flat, heart-shaped seed pods and is similar to the peppergrasses. The basal leaves are dandelionlike, while the stem leaves are clasping. It produces white flowers that are found on spikelike clusters. Shepherd's purse flowers from mid-spring to mid-fall, and is found throughout the United States.

Personality   Oddly enough, the one and only plant I learned about during my short stint with the Boy Scouts was shepherd's purse. My brother Jim and I were both patrol leaders and were chosen to explore areas of the Pine Barrens in search of a place to hold one of the many summer campouts. Rick and I eventually quit the Boy Scout movement because we could not stand staying in tents and cooking canned foods, or for that matter, the regimented requirements during these campouts. Though I believe that the Boy Scout movement is very important for today's youth, it wasn't for the well-trained survivalists Rick and I were. However, I do feel that the basic training the Boy Scouts offer today is very important to a person's life and bolsters his awareness of the natural world and his respect for it.

Jim and I had been traveling most of the day, stopping at various spots to check out the potential camps. It had taken far longer than anticipated, and we were without food, water, or shelter of any sort. At one of the resting places, Jim identified a plant called shepherd's purse, which the Scout manual said was edible. Grandfather had said nothing of this plant even though we had passed it several times during our travels, so I was rather skeptical as to its edibility. So many things taught in the Boy Scout manual were barely adequate, especially in the survival section where some were complete failures under certain conditions. I was not about to trust any book fully, and I had a high respect for plants.

After a few minutes of argument, and settling on the fact that the Scout fathers would not put plants in the manual that would hurt us, we decided to try it. Our hunger at that point far surpassed clear thinking and caution, at any rate. Furthermore, in the few campouts we had taken with the Scouts, Rick and I were the only ones to ever try the edible plants and camp in a semisurvival condition. We were looked on as mavericks but most of the Scouts wanted to become members of our rebel patrol. My brother, being cautious, allowed me to prepare the shepherd's purse since at that time he hadn't ever eaten any of the natural plants. He was also smart enough to allow

185

me to eat the plant first as soon as it was prepared.

I cooked up the leaves like spinach and cautiously sampled the herb. It was delicious and I quickly ate the whole bowl. Then I decided to munch on a few of the more succulent fresh leaves, which turned out to be just as delicious. Jim watched me as if I were about to keel over with an exotic case of plant poisoning at any moment. After what seemed to be a long while, he also sampled the plant and quickly finished the bowl. Another batch was prepared until we were full. From that point on, any time Jim and I entered the woods for the Boy Scouts or for exploration, he would get me to teach him new plants. Finally he turned his patrol into a survival-camping patrol as Rick and I had done.

It is sad because, in a way, Jim and I began to come together closer than any two brothers ever had. Even though I left the Scouts, Jim never held it against me, and we still continued our mutual explorations of the wilderness areas and all the survival techniques. Jim had shown great promise as an outdoorsman and easily blended with the Earth until he received a bad ankle injury during a fifty-mile hike on a Scout reservation. The result was a long series of operations, casts on his leg for many months, and a long period away from the woods and school. Once the cast was off, he could no longer take long hikes abroad so his interest turned to other things. For a long time I felt a great loss. He had been a companion in exploration who could no longer come with me, and I felt as if I had been robbed of one of my best friends. It wasn't until just a few years ago that he regained his ability to hike long distances and soon we will be wandering again.

I would not let Jim's injury stand in the way of his savoring wilderness and edible plants. We would spend countless hours near the house, contentedly exploring and sampling the little things in the immediate area. Many times after a long hike, I would bring plants back to the house for him to sample. I've always admired his tenacity and dedication to learning even during the times all odds were against him. In many ways, his dedication and discipline have been guiding forces in my life. I really don't think that Jim and I would have ever known each other as well as we did if it weren't for the first plant we sampled on our own. Every time I pass a shepherd's purse, I think of my brother, and even though we are worlds apart in our professions, we have a common bond to wilderness and each other through that plant.

Jim and I, in a joint effort, attempted to bring the wild edible plants to our home's dinner table. The first dish we prepared for a

Scout banquet was made from shepherd's purse and was a big hit. We cooked up the greens like spinach and garnished them with the seeds of the shepherd, which adds a great peppery taste. We also created a wild edible salad, made mostly of succulent shepherd's purse leaves, and garnished with homemade Italian dressing with the plant's peppery seeds. We were both delighted at the outcome, and under the influence of Jim, Rick, and me, the whole troop moved toward a deeper and closer understanding of the Earth. Today, Jim is still involved in the Boy Scout movement and has led many troops back to the Earth and the excitement of camping in a real way.

Food   The heart-shaped seeds of shepherd's purse can be collected in late summer and early fall. They should be dried in the mellow sun over a few days. Be careful to put them out late and bring them in early so as to avoid the settling of dew. I grind the seeds into a coarse powder, store it in an old pepper shaker, and use it as a pepper substitute. I keep whole seeds or those only lightly ground for salad dressings and other foods where pepper bits are merited. I am sure anyone would enjoy the unique taste of these seeds more than the usual common black pepper.

The young leaves, gathered before the plant flowers, can be cooked like spinach by simmering in water for ten to fifteen minutes. The fresh young leaves can also be added raw to salads or used as a garnish on many different plates. As the plant flowers and begins to develop seeds, the leaves turn slightly coarse and bitter. This can be easily taken care of by boiling for fifteen to twenty minutes in two consecutive changes of water. The older leaves take a little getting used to and become more of an acquired taste. Usually, if you are an avid herbalist and like the stronger wild edibles as I do, you will find the older leaves more suitable to your tastes and will begin to prefer them over the younger leaves.

Medicinal   During one of my survival campouts, I got a bad cut across my knee, which would not stop bleeding. I had fallen onto a piece of gravel with a sharp edge and the wound was jagged and deep. It definitely needed stitches. Grandfather prepared a strong tea by using the leaves of shepherd's purse and steeped it for about fifteen minutes. He allowed it to cool then used it to wash my cut thoroughly. Within a few moments, the bleeding had slowed down, and a short time later, it had completely stopped. I was truly amazed at the coagulant effect of the tea on the bleeding. Later on in my career, I found that the tea made from shepherd's purse has an ability to constrict blood vessels.

I have also seen Grandfather use this tea to control people's high blood pressure. Even though it tends to constrict the blood vessels, it usually works in an emergency situation to control either high or low blood pressure. One of Grandfather's patients who had problems with high blood pressure used the tea faithfully to control the problem. Once his blood pressure came down, his frequent headaches disappeared. For an all-around tonic, Grandfather would mix a small palmful of fresh herb or two small palmfuls of dried herb with one-half cup of water and steep for fifteen minutes. The dose was taken one cup every other day, a little at a time, for a week, then discontinued.

The tea can also stimulate bowel movement, and in some people eliminate excess water retention. A strong tea makes a good antiseptic and aids blood coagulation. The dried herb must never be kept for more than two seasons as it quickly loses its medicinal qualities and begins to break down. It is best stored in an earthenware container in a cool place. Drying time should be slow and with good air circulation so as to retain most of the plant's medicinal qualities during drying.

Warning: *In some people, the tea can elevate high blood pressure instead of lowering it. I would not recommend the use of this herb as a blood pressure remedy unless in a survival situation where no modern alternatives are present.*

Spicebush (*Lindera benzoin*)

Description   Spicebush is a low spicy-scented shrub found in damp woods, streamsides, and other damp areas. The leaves are thin and elliptical, toothless and hairless, and richly aromatic. The bark of the tree is smooth, and the twigs are slim and very brittle at most times of the year. The spicy-scented yellowish flowers erupt before the leaves of spring, and the fruits are deep red, oval, and contain a single seed. They are found throughout the eastern United States, from Canada south to Missouri and North Carolina. Spicebush is found from Maine, to Michigan and adjacent Canada.

Personality   In his daily teachings, Grandfather tried to stimulate our interest by creating mysteries. These mysteries would add a sense of excitement to our learning experience and fire our interest far more than school ever did. Learning with Grandfather was always fun, always interesting, and what he wanted to teach us was always something we wanted to know. Grandfather used to create the problems, then nearly lead us to the answers before turning us loose. The learning process was a series of trials and errors, hints and frustrations, all designed to give us experience in problem solving and in the mistakes surrounding a skill.

Spicebush was no exception to the rule of the mystery learning that Grandfather called "coyote teaching." It began with a cup of tea and, after a long search for answers, ended a year later with another cup of tea. The tea was first tasted during a mid-winter campout on a very cold night. We had just returned from a foraging trip into a small swamp and were literally chilled to the bone. The fire was of no help so Grandfather prepared us a cup of tea. The tea was delicious, warming, and had a taste we had never experienced before. Not only did it taste good but it smelled even better, enticing our senses and, of course, our curiosity.

Grandfather was sketchy with his information about the origin of the tea. He said that the tea came from a small tree that could be found at the northern edge of the Pine Barrens but the origins were vague at best. The rest, he said, would have to come from our own exploration, and the smell should be enough to help us locate this mysterious tea. Not even sassafras could come close to the delicious smells of this mystery tree, but sassafras was the closest thing we had to its identity. We savored the next cup of this mystery tea for almost an hour, trying to make the taste and smell part of our memory so we would know the tree when we came upon it.

Every time we went to the northern edge of the Pine Barrens we would test the various trees we didn't know. Even the ones we knew quite well were thoroughly examined and smelled as we tried desperately to find the missing piece of the puzzle. Months went by, but time was not enough to quench our persistent search and curiosity. Grandfather, too, would drop hints and reminders to keep us alert to all the trees and to our quest to solve the mystery. There was never a trip to the northern Barrens that we did not spend half our time looking for that elusive tree. We even revisited trees that we had scrutinized in other seasons, hoping that their scent had changed to what we were looking for.

During the winter following the tree mystery, we were back in the same area of the northern Barrens where we had tasted the tea for the first time. Rick was tending the fire and I was leaning back against a small tree, sinew-wrapping a fletch on one of my arrows. Grandfather was busy making a tea near a small fire just outside his debris hut. The aroma of the tea hit Rick and me almost simultaneously and we knew instantly that Grandfather was brewing the mystery tea. To help myself up faster, I grabbed hold of a small branch of the young tree and began to pull myself up. The branch snapped and I fell on my backside, feeling a little embarrassed. We drank the tea, savoring its essence and mildly complaining that it had been almost a year since we first tasted the tea but still had no clue to what it was.

Grandfather laughed and admonished us that we were looking too hard and making the matter too complicated. I retreated back to my arrow wrapping, pondering what Grandfather had said, trying to figure out what he meant. For hours as I sat doing camp chores, I could still smell the tea. The scent was so fresh in the air it was as if it were just being brewed again. I intermittently looked over at Grandfather's camp to see if he were actually brewing the tea, only to find him doing other things. That was when I saw a leaf fall and it dawned on me which way the wind was blowing. Even if Grandfather were brewing tea, the essence could not be carried upwind.

I searched the area frantically for the origin of the scent. At first, I thought it was the residual left in my cup but that was downwind, too. I looked all around but saw nothing out of the ordinary. Frustrated I sat back down to do some work. Out of the corner of my eye I caught sight of the broken branch and felt compelled to smell the break. The shouting that ensued flooded the camp. Rick picked up his club and began swinging as if we were being attacked by wild dogs. Grandfather fell on the ground, laughing so hard that he could not get up. I ran around jumping and singing that I had found the answer to the mystery. To an outsider, the whole affair would have looked serious enough to commit us to some rest home.

Ironically, we learned the valuable lesson of trying too hard. We also learned not to assume or try to second-guess anything. We had assumed that the tree was in the distant north and that Grandfather would never give us a problem so simple that the answer would be right under our noses. If we had not been so caught up in our own prejudicial thoughts as to where we thought the tree would be, then we would have searched the immediate area first. Instead, because of some preconceived idea, we decided that the tree was in a different place than where we had originally tasted it. Our prejudice also precluded any new thought or direction. This lesson taught us quite a bit about the way our minds can cause us to think a feeling instead of really feeling it.

Food   Since that day we learned about spicebush after a year of searching, we learned much more about its uses. The tree provided teas year-round, each season and part producing its own unique tea with a distinct flavor. In fall and winter, we could make a rich tea from the tender twigs and tips. In the spring and summer we would use the new fresh leaves for a milder tea. It was best to use the tree fresh, but we also had great success with the dried leaves and smaller twigs. The drying process was like any other except it was done slower so that the leaves or twigs did not lose their flavor. In fall or spring, we would gather the twigs, scrape off the bark, and dry the scrapings. In spring and summer we would collect only the newest and most tender leaves for drying, thus producing an excellent stash. For dried tea we would mix equal parts bark scrapings and leaves to get the best brew.

Grandmother was instrumental in teaching us the other uses of spicebush. We joined her in the field one warm, later summer afternoon to help her with her herbal collection for the winter months. We collected various herbs, roots, tubers, nuts, and berries for several hours, finally stopping at a small grove of spicebush. Their deep red berries shone from the delicate greens of the leaves like jewels, much like holly. We collected the berries for over an hour, not knowing what Grandmother was going to do with them. We knew about the tea but had no idea if we could also use the berries. When we asked Grandmother, she said that we should not eat the berries for they can be poisonous unless prepared properly, and she would show us how to use them when we got back to her home.

We spent several hours that night cutting up the small berries and removing the seed. The seeds were placed in a small container and would not be used except for replanting in the spring. The fleshy berry part was what Grandmother was interested in. The next day we dried all the berries in the hot sun, then spent much of the night grinding them with a simple mortar and pestel into a fine granular powder. Grandmother then told us many stories about spicebush. It was used by our pioneer ancestors as a substitute for allspice. She cautioned us that it should be used sparingly as a spice and not eaten in great quantities. I have come to prefer spicebush as an alternative to allspice in all my recipes requiring allspice.

Medicinal I have effectively used spicebush as a wash for mild skin irritations and wounds. For afflictions such as poison ivy or insect stings, I brew a stronger tea made from the rootbark. It must be remembered that this is only a mild skin wash and other plants should be substituted when a stronger remedy is required. I find the wash especially useful for people who have sensitive skin.

Sumac (*Rhus spp.*—except *Rhus vernix*)

Description   Sumacs are small trees or shrubs with large compound leaves. The twigs are very thick and pithy with a milky sap. The fruit clusters are red and hairy and usually found at the end of branches. These clusters can persist well into the winter. Depending on species, the leaves can be toothed or toothless. They are lovers of waste grounds, old fields, and fence roads. One or more species are found throughout the United States.

Personality   My first baptism into the world of sumac was utilitarian. It began with experiments with the various woods and herbacius stalks that could be used to make our bow drill apparatus. We then found that the pithy centers of the stalks could be easily burned out, producing great pipe stems and blowguns. Our blowguns were never used for hunting but mostly for target practice and attempts at duplicating the precision the jungle people of South America possessed. Another encounter with sumac was with the poison sumac, which produced a horrid rash that persisted for over two weeks and was more painful than the worse case of poison ivy I ever had. You can bet we learned quickly to tell the difference between poison sumac and its usable relatives.

Sumac is a grand survival utilitarian plant, and we used it for quite some time before we ever learned of its edibility. During one late summer outing, we discovered the first edible use of the sumac, part through accident and part through Grandfather. We were collecting a sumac stem to be used for a blowgun. It was custom that we buried the red-seeded heads so that they would take root. While doing this I inadvertently got some of the sticky parts on my hands. A little later on, I wiped the sweat from my face and got some of the sticky liquid on my lips. Licking my lips, I found that the juice had a bit of a citric taste, which I immediately asked Grandfather about. I was more in fear of possibly dying from some strange plant poisoning rather than finding out if it were edible or not.

Grandfather had us gather a few flowerheads, and he placed them into a container of ice-cold water that he got from a nearby stream. He gently broke up the heads, rubbing the seeds between his palms. He let this concoction settle for about a half hour then strained it through a grass sieve. We cautiously tasted the cool liquid and found, to our delight, that it tasted much like lemonade. It was just as refreshing to me, and I preferred it over either iced tea or lemonade. Sumac became one of our standard summer drinks that we would drink hot or cold.

Grandmother made a delicious combination of iced teas using sumac, mint, and store-bought tea. She would mix these in equal parts, sweeten with honey, and add lemon. It was a thirst-quenching, cool summer drink that we enjoyed anytime we passed Grandmother's house. My only bad experience with sumac tea was when I didn't take enough care in the filtering and preparation, allowing the small hairs and parts of berries to get into my drink. The sensation of the gritty hair particles in my throat and mouth was quite uncomfortable and took many drinks of fresh water to wash out.

The first medicinal use of sumac I discovered during the winter months when I had a sore throat and cold sores from the backlash of a common cold. Grandfather prepared a tea, using the bark of a young stalk. I used it as a gargle. The sore throat disappeared and I felt an astonishing relief of the cold sore pain. He then took a small sumac root, washed and scraped it, then told me to chew on it periodically throughout the day. This had a marvelous effect on my cold sores and soothed the pain. They disappeared in half the time that it would normally have taken. A few weeks later the same bark tea was used to treat Rick for a bad case of diarrhea. The results again were quick and effective with absolutely no side effects or the constipation that usually follows the use of modern medications for diarrhea.

Food The mature sumac berry heads contain numerous acidic hairs. Collect the berry clusters when they are red and ripe, before the heavy rains wash away the acidic properties. Place the heads in cold water and lightly bruise between palms. Allow to soak from ten to fifteen minutes. Remove the flowerheads and strain the remaining liquid through a grass filter or cheesecloth. This will effectively remove any residual berries and the hairs. Some people prefer to sweeten the drink, but I prefer mine as is. You may find that you will begin to prefer the sumac drink over all other typical commercial summer drinks. I have used the berry heads long past prime, and though many more are needed, you can still produce a fine drink. Take care not to remove too many, as many song birds and other wildlife use the berries as winter food.

Warning: *Do not confuse the edible sumacs with the poisonous sumac. The poison sumac has loose, white berries and can cause dermatitis far worse than poison ivy. I suggest very strongly that you consult a good field guide for proper identification and comparison.*

Medicinal   A tea can be made from the bark, new leaves, and ripe berries, singularly or in combination. Steep a palmful of bark, berries, or leaves in one cup of cold water from thirty to forty-five minutes depending on the strength of the tea needed. The tea should be taken in the dosage of one to two cups a day, one-quarter cup at a time. It can be used as a gargle for sore throat or cold sores. It can also be used to abate diarrhea and for urinary problems. For urinary problems it is best to use the leaves. Milder teas come from the berries, stronger teas from the leaves, and the strongest from the roots. The sumac roots can be chewed periodically for cold sores, but don't overdo it, as too much can have adverse effects.

A poultice of pounded seedheads and fresh leaves makes a good remedy for poison ivy. For a stronger poison ivy medication, you can boil roots, leaves, and seedheads into a strong tea and use as a general skin wash or to stop bleeding. The best for the stoppage of bleeding of minor skin abrasions is a mild tea made from the berries, steeped in warm water for a few minutes. A thick warm tea, made from the seedheads, simmered almost to a syruplike consistency, is great for reducing fever and for other mouth irritations.

Warning: *Some people are allergic to the bark, roots, and leaves of the sumac, so use sparingly the first time.*

Sweet Fern (*Comptonia peregrina*)

Description   Sweet fern is a low bush, deciduous, with fern-like leaves bearing a nutlike fruit that is not waxy. It is a lover of dry or sandy soils and is found from the Canadian border, south to Virginia and northeast Illinois. It may also range into Minnesota.

Personality   On our more advanced campouts in the fall, my students take a special liking to sweet fern. It grows quite extensively throughout the Pine Barrens and is one of the more accessible and easily found wild edible plants. To the beginning students cast into a full survival situation after only a week of intense instruction, the diet at first is usually very bland. Once we introduce them to sweet fern, the students tend to favor this plant over all other available ones. It is a delicious tea with a distinctive taste. Blended with wintergreen, which also grows in the same areas, it is a welcome treat for the students. Many of the students take to planting this little herb on their own, some even take the seeds home with them to try and plant them indoors. Besides being delicious, it makes a beautiful house plant when properly cared for. It has become very popular with my western students, who can't easily get it in their area, that they ask me to send them dried leaves. It becomes one of their cherished favorites.

My students are interested in everything involving nature. So anytime there is a new use for a plant, they flock to see what they can pick up. One of the students had a serious problem with a case of poison ivy that would not go away. Even though he became infected a few days earlier at his home, it continued to persist well into our survival campout. I had one of the students gather up a bunch of the leaves and bring them back to camp where one of my instructors prepared them. He finely chopped the leaves, then simmered them into a very strong tea for over half an hour. I had the student wash all the calamine lotion from his body, as he looked like he was composed totally of the hardened pink lotion. I felt that medication would not work well with the interference of the calamine lotion.

He wiped on the tea while it was still warm, bathing all the affected areas two and three times. Within a few minutes the intense itching stopped. We repeated the application several times during the day until the swelling and oozing disappeared. By the morning of the next day, most of the redness and all of the itching had disappeared. My students were amazed that there was such a dramatic recovery. Many of them believed, as most people do, that herbal remedies are mild at best or mere superstition. They could not believe that this student, who had tried most poison ivy remedies as well as taking drugs internally, would respond so well to a natural remedy. Respond he did so that by the end of two days, all traces of the poison ivy was gone, except the scars and scabs left from his scratching.

To Grandfather, sweet fern was more than a good tea. He would use it throughout the winter. He spoke highly of the plant to all his patients and encouraged them to store their own stash for the winter months. It was not uncommon to see several of the older people and a few herbalists out on a sunny summer morning gathering up the herb while intermittently planting the seeds. We would always help Grandfather with his collecting, not only because he had to supply so many people, but we wanted to collect our own stash. We loved to listen to his stories and songs as he collected, always reverent to the plant people that meant so much to him. Not only was there the power of the sweet fern alone, but it also served as a catalyst for so many other medicinal mixtures and compounds.

We would take our collection of leaves, sort through them for any damage or insect scars, then lay them out to dry in the mild sun. Once the leaves became brittle, but still containing some of their green color, they were ready for preparation. We would then meticulously break them up into a tealike consistency, and wrap them in small cheesecloth bags. We would then hang them in a cool dry place for about a week until they were finally transferred into earthenware or glass containers. Each batch was watched carefully by Grandfather. The smaller leaves would be used as tea and the older leaves used as catalysts and stronger teas.

At the end of the day, we would take some of the newly dried smaller leaves and brew up a mild tea. Relaxing, talking, or telling stories, we would sip our tea well into the night, thanking the Creator for such a powerful brother. The sweet fern taught us much about the different tastes and powers of plants during various times of the season. We learned the various tastes and powers of the new plants, the older plants with new and old leaves, and plants growing in certain areas compared to others growing in other areas. They were remarkably different. It was subtle, but we could even tell if the leaves were collected before, during, or after a rain, and even what part of the forest a certain plant grew, just from the taste of its tea.

We learned to mix the various parts of the sweet fern. New leaves from one region were mixed with older leaves from another, producing a subtle but different taste to the tea. Watching Grandfather administer the tea to the various people also taught us that different parts of the plant needed to be used on different patients. He always seemed to get the right plant part and the proper mixture. His favorite was mixing tiny leaves of wintergreen with the older leaves of sweet fern, steeping them for one hour in cold water then heating the mixture up. This tea was one of the better tonic teas especially when a person was close to getting a cold. Rose hips were added to this mixture for people who already had colds.

The first time I really saw the wonders of sweet fern work as a medicine was when a friend of mine had a badly swollen boil. My friend was visiting for the weekend and the boil restricted his movement and was otherwise painful. On our way to the swimming hole, we came upon Grandfather and I told him of my friend's plight, much to my friend's embarrassment. Grandfather gathered some green sweet fern, mashed them in water until it appeared as equal parts water and herb, and simmered it into a thick poultice. Placing the warm poultice on the boil until it cooled, he repeated the process three times. Upon removal of the final compress, the boil had ruptured and was draining well. Grandfather wiped the area clean with a milder sweet fern tea, and my friend was no longer bothered by the pain all weekend. It disappeared the following day.

Food Sweet fern makes some of the finest teas I have ever tasted. It also blends beautifully with other natural and cultivated teas to make a unique and stimulating blend. The teas should be made from slowly dried leaves (leaves dried in a cool, dry place). Green leaves have a more medicinal value and should not be used. Older leaves make the strongest tea, younger leaves a mild tea, and the first new succulent leaves of spring make a milder tea yet, which is my favorite. Sweet fern tea can be mixed with equal parts of any other tea. Wintergreen, pine, mint, catnip, yarrow, and birch are some of my favorite mixes. Sweet fern tea can also be served cold and sweetened with honey to your liking.

Medicinal A strong cup of tea made from the partially dried leaves is good for stopping diarrhea and relieving cramps. The tea should be made by taking a good palmful of leaves and soaking in warm water for forty-five minutes. An even stronger tea can be used for a mouthwash for gum disorders or other wounds of the mouth. The strong tea made from the entire plant, or a poultice made from the green leaves, can be used for a skin wash. It has astringent properties which alleviate poison ivy, bee stings, sunburn, and other skin ailments. I have also used it effectively on my children's acne.

Many of the older folks of my neighborhood used the stronger sweet fern teas as a tonic. They would take one-half cup a day, every other day. Many of them swear that it keeps their bowel movement regular and is good for warding off common colds. Other people use the pulverized leaves as a toothpaste, and a stronger tea as a mouthwash. Be careful when carrying around the whole leaves as they look, to the untrained eye, like marijuana. Some of my students have been arrested for possession of these leaves, which were carried in a plastic bag, only to be released later on by a rather embarrassed police department.

Thistle (*Cirsium spp.*)

Description   Thistles love sunny pastures, abandoned farm fields, and roadsides. Stems are erect and prickly with yellow-tipped spines on the bracts. The flowerheads are large and shaped much like shaving brushes. They come in rose, purple, pink, or red. The leaves are prickly and deeply cut. The plant produces a rosette the first year, and the flowers spike or stalk in the second year. One or more species can be found throughout the country.

Personality   I come from a very Scottish background. My father moved to this country just after World War II from Glasgow, Scotland, and my mother is of full Scottish ancestry. My very first recollection of the thistle plant was when I was quite young and my father told stories of his homeland. The thistle is the national flower of Scotland and it comes with a very proud past. According to legend, it saved the Scottish army during its fight with the English army. Apparently, the English army tried to sneak up on the Scottish army during one of their wars and, as the Roman armies had done many years before, ran into a bed of thistle. The screams of pain alerted the Scottish army, and they were not taken by surprise. Thus the thistle saved many lives and helped win an important battle.

My respect for the plant grew much stronger every time I would venture out with my dad to pick the fine thistle flowers. No matter how careful I was in the collection, I always came away looking as if I, too, had just lost a battle. I felt a certain kinship to the British armies and how they felt when marching through the legions of tenacious thistle. I certainly began to respect the thistle for its beauty and its history, as well as for the wounds it could easily inflict on a less-than-careful boy.

My first real lesson with the thistle came when Grandfather and I were exploring the upper reaches of the Toms River, near Jackson. We had to go a long distance over a route that had no streams or ponds. We lovingly called this route the dry route because it was many miles and hours before we could get any water. We also reserved our travel over this route to the cooler months, when water was not as critical. This time we took the route in mid-August on a hot, dry, and dusty day. Before half the trip was over, I thought that I was surely going to die of thirst. Complaints from Rick and me continued until we entered a huge field.

The field was a gorgeous collection of greenery and rafts of wildflowers of every description. It was one big pasture for all the insects and birds that seek the nectar of flowers, and was so strikingly beautiful and full of life that we wanted to rest here and explore. For hours we wandered in the sun, studying wildflowers, animal trails, old bird nests, and hundreds of other things. We were so enraptured in the magic of the field that we abandoned all thought of bodily comfort. Our minds were so caught up in the tremendous beauty that our concentration propelled us into the eternity of the moment. As we were about to leave, however, all the pain of thirst, sunburn, and fatigue returned, this time with a vengeance.

Grandfather also seemed hot and thirsty, though it was hard to tell with him because he always looked so mellow and at peace. He seemed to blend in wherever he was, becoming one with the land-scape, as if he belonged there. We followed him to the edge of the field where he motioned for us to sit down. Approaching a huge bull thistle, he cut off one of the larger center leaves, uttering a small inaudible prayer as he took it. Carefully, he took his knife and peeled off all the thorns, then gave it a once-over with the edge of the blade to insure all the spines were gone. The result was a clean leafstalk that looked very similar to celery.

He began to eat this stalk, much as we would have eaten a stalk of celery. With each bite, we could see a mist of water expelled. He motioned for us to take some of the thistle plants, explaining that they would temporarily quench our thirst, as they primarily were made up of water. We were a bit cautious, taking extra care to make sure all the spines were removed. There was something a bit scary about chomping down on a plant that under natural conditions could inflict tremendous pain. The taste was not unlike celery, though a little wilder. Our thirsts were quenched, and in the process of ob-taining water from the plant, we were also eating lunch. We were truly amazed that such a tenacious plant on the outside could be so soothing and helpful to us in a survival situation.

Our lessons of the thistle were far from over for there were still so many ways we could use the plant. Through the fall, we learned to use its dethorned stalk as a hand drill, its downy seeds parachute as a tinder-bundle additive. However, approaching the colder part of the winter, we learned and appreciated much more about the plant. Food on our winter survival outing was scarce. We were camped near the thistle field, and in that area of the Barrens, most of the edibles had gone to seed or their roots were frozen in the ground. We were very hungry and our traps produced little due to the adverse cold and windy weather. Animals seemed to be hiding, as if afraid to come out. We wondered what we were doing outside.

Grandfather walked into the field with us. I thought that he was going to set a trap with the way he looked at the ground. He searched various areas until he stopped at a certain location and looked down. There at his feet was the withering remains of a thistle rosette, still containing a bit of green despite the cold. He easily dug the root from the ground with a sharp stick. He peeled it then broke it into three parts, giving us each one. We ate these to placate our appetites as we went about gathering other roots from various rosettes, taking care to leave enough for the next season. These were cooked and eaten much like carrots. They were absolutely delicious and filling, to say the least. We welcomed the addition to our meager diets and ate until we could hardly walk.

Food   The new pithy stems of spring can be peeled and eaten raw or cooked like a green. I prefer a quick cooking or a steaming as you would prepare asparagus. The young leaves can be peeled of their spines and cooked in the same way as the young stems, eaten raw, or added to salads. Older leaves are a bit more bitter, but I prefer their taste, either cooked or raw, to the other parts of the plant. To get rid of the slight bitterness and stringy texture, older leaves can be boiled in two changes of water for ten minutes. The roots of the first-year rosettes are excellent peeled and eaten raw or cooked. They can be used throughout the fall and winter and are a source of emergency survival food that is quite nourishing.

Medicinal   For medicinal purposes, the roots can be used dry or fresh. Fresh roots produce the best medicinal value, although dried roots are recommended for use by people with sensitive skin. Simmer a good palmful of roots in one pint of water for forty minutes. While simmering, crush the roots so that as much root fiber as possible is exposed to the hot water. Strain the liquid. The remaining root poultice can be applied directly to boils, insect stings, poison ivy, or ulcerated areas of the body. The strong tea can be used as a mouth wash for cold sores or gum problems or can be used as an effective skin wash for infections. Use chilled to abate the itch of poison ivy or other itchy patches of skin.

Violet (*Viola spp.*)

Description   Most of the violet species love wet meadows, damp woods, and generally moist conditions. However, the birdfoot violet prefers sandy and sunny areas. The violet is one of our familiar spring flowers. Its flowers can be blue-violet, yellow, or white, and have five petals, with the lowest petal extending back into a spur. This petal is usually heavily veined, whereas the lateral petals are usually bearded. These flower shapes can vary according to species. Generally, the leaves of the violet are heart shaped, except for the birdfoot violet whose leaves resemble that of a bird's foot. One or more species can be found from Maine, west to North Dakota and adjacent Canada, and south to the Gulf of Mexico.

Personality   Violets were one of my most powerful spiritual teachers in the area of inner awareness and communication. At the time, I knew nothing of the violets other than what they looked like and their name. They weren't found directly in my area but to the more northwestern areas of the Pine Barrens. Grandfather had never really mentioned the violet because there were so many other plants we had to learn. We did admire its beauty, stopping to scrutinize the plant closely whenever we saw them. Their flowers were gorgeous and the leaves succulent, especially in the early spring when there wasn't much competition among the plants.

It was at this time that Grandfather was trying to teach us to nurture the inner voice, gut instinct, or spiritual communication. It was a difficult concept for young boys, but we began to sense things on deeper levels as our teachings progressed. Many times I would hear Grandfather say that a camp area didn't "feel good" to him and we would go on to another. Later we would learn that a wild dog pack had run through or a beer party had taken place near the area. Grandfather's sixth sense, his inner awareness, was uncanny at times, allowing him to see deeper into things than we could ever imagine.

These gut instincts and communications were of utmost importance to anyone who lived for long periods of time in the wilderness. They were just as important as the shelter, bow drill, or the gathering of water. They helped the tracker and survivalist see beyond the physical senses and into a world of the "spirits" as he called them. To him, and to us, there was a world out there that the ancients spoke of often. This was the world of spirituality that could only be reached through the heart and not with the mind. Grandfather's most difficult chore was to teach us to shut down our doubting minds and listen to the voices of Creation with our hearts. Shutting out the petty doubts and worries was a major task, mainly because I was so full of energy and wonder.

As the years passed, we grew very adept at picking out the tiny voices and nuances of the landscape. We would somehow know something without any real logical explanation as to why. We began to accept these things without question as we relied more and more on our gut feelings and listened with our hearts. We probed and explored beyond the normal world of physical sight and sound and saw deeper into even the most common entities, a world that no one else seemed to pay attention to. We perceived the Earth as a living being and all things of the Earth as profound teachers, not only in the physical sense but also in spiritual realms.

One day when we were sitting by a small stream at the western edge of the Pine Barrens, Grandfather handed me a plant. Close inspection showed me that it was a violet that he had picked near the edge of the stream. I smiled up at him and told him that it was a violet, feeling very confident about my identification. He asked me what else I could tell him about it, and I had to say that I didn't know much about it but its name. He then told me to ask it to reveal its inner secrets, explaining that the plants and animals could teach me far more than any books or logical analysis. I was taken aback by his words and had no idea of what he was talking about or even how to go about asking the plant anything. I suspected it did have something to do with the inner voice and listening with our hearts.

I stared blankly at the plant, feeling foolish that I could not see anything that would reveal any secrets. Grandfather said, "Look with your heart: You look but do not see, you listen but do not hear, you taste but do not savor, and you touch but do not feel. Let your mind and physical senses go and reach out with your true inner feelings so that you become one with the spirit of the plant." I was trying as hard as I could to shut down my mind and senses, but it was no use, the plant just felt like a plant and I could not feel what Grandfather asked.

We abandoned the subject and continued our rest. Rick explored the outer areas of the deciduous forest, Grandfather walked upstream, and I wrote in my notebook. When we all came back together to resume our trip, Grandfather caught me nibbling on something and coyly asked me what it was. I pulled the partially eaten plant from my mouth and to my shock it was part of the violet. He then asked me where the rest of the plants he had picked had gone. Shocked, I said that I must have eaten them. He smiled with utter delight and told me that the plant had communicated with me on a deeper level and that it took the distraction of writing in my journal to bring it out.

Sure enough, the plant was edible and quite delicious. It took me years to piece back together the chain of events that led up to my eating those plants. I realize now that it was my logical mind and the logical belief that the world of the spirits do not exist that kept me from communicating with the plant. I understood many things about that plant through intuition which I could have never learned from a book, and to this day, one of my biggest quests is to cultivate this inner awareness with all things. This is critical if one is to ever be a good survivalist, tracker, naturalist, or especially an herbalist. The cultivation of that inner voice, that communication, and that awareness are the most important skills.

Food   I have always used the violet as a trailside nibble. Both the flowers and the new leaves I find absolutely delicious. Some people do not like the plain violet greens but prefer them mixed with other greens in a salad. I find that the more a person eats the wild edibles, the more he or she likes the greens alone. The greens and flowers can also be steamed for ten minutes or cooked like spinach by simmering them in hot water for ten minutes. Experiment with the cooking of violets because the length of cooking time has great bearing on their taste.

I dry the new leaves and flowers in a cool dry place for several hours then store them in earthenware containers or buckskin bags. I find that violet tea is very delicious alone or mixed with other teas. Some old-timers prefer violet tea mixed fifty-fifty with Oriental or strawberry teas, and used as a tonic. Some of my students also prefer violet tea chilled as an iced-tea substitute. Grandfather made a delicious tea by steeping the fresh flowers in hot water for one-half hour. Violet leaves are rich in vitamin C.

Warning: *Most members of the violet family are edible. However, some of the yellow species may have a mild, cathartic effect.*

Medicinal   The violet is not a strong medicine by itself, but it greatly enhances other medicinal teas, medicines, and compounds as a catalyst. Grandpa Dandelion used to make a tonic out of violet tea by mixing with other teas in equal parts. Violet tea was mixed with alfalfa, sweet yellow clover, birch, mint, catnip, and rose hips. During the cold season, he would also mix in a little yarrow leaves and, of course, tea made from dandelion greens. I didn't like the taste, but I loved the power of that tea as a general tonic.

Wintergreen (*Gaultheria procumbens*)

Description Wintergreen loves poor soils in the woods or clearings. They grow close to the ground on long interconnecting root systems. The leaves are oval, slightly toothed, shiny, and thick. It is an evergreen with tiny white, waxy flowers that dangle underneath the little umbrella of leaves. It flowers throughout the summer, and the berries can be found from late summer to the next early summer. Wintergreen grows from Canada and the northern United States to as far south as Georgia, following the mountain ranges.

Personality Wintergreen has always been one of my favorites, mostly because it is always there when you need it either for a medication or a food. Wintergreen was one of my earliest plant acquaintances and I never tire of its companionship. In the spring and summer, it appears to be a little umbrella of green, hugging the ground close, as if loving the Earth. We would lie on our bellies, relaxing after a long hike and imagine the tiny animals that would take refuge from the sun beneath the leaves. To us, this little plant was truly an Earth plant, and in fact, the first name I remember calling this little plant is Earth plant. In the fall, we would find the little berries, and during the winter months, beneath the melting snow, we could still find the elegant greenery. The plant seemed totally unaffected by weather. For its size, it had a tenacious personality.

Our travels when we were very young were limited to the forest between Rick's house and mine. It wasn't a big area, possibly a half mile long and about the same in width, but rarely did anyone go there. At its outer edges was a continuous thick and hardy wall of brier bushes, and very few children would venture through it, never any adults. There we had our little pretend camp, fashioned from the forest and bits that society had cast off. Survival to us at that time was but a dream, and it was more make-believe than hard skill. What few skills we did learn, we practiced frequently in this world built between imagination and reality. Every tidbit of knowledge that Grandfather passed out was cherished by us.

Our camp was made up of a two-boy debris hut (making it was one of the skills we first learned), a fire pit, a low table made from an old piece of plywood, numerous stumps for sitting, old rope, caches, and a few cans of emergency food. Our latest project was learning the bow-drill fire-making method, and we were also experimenting with collecting water. This was our true home, a place to relax, break rules, and enjoy the natural world that intrigued both of us. Any time

Grandfather came to visit, it was like a festive holiday. We would prepare our camp for days in advance so everything was tidy and blended into the natural landscape.

Grandfather was a coyote teacher and taught us more by leading us toward a truth and stimulating intense interest, than by actually showing us anything. Frequently, our learning was by trial and error as we put together the bits and pieces of what Grandfather had given us. From these fragments, we would build our skills and also the experience that only trial and error can build. We thirsted for knowledge and watched Grandfather carefully, never knowing when he was going to give us a clue. We had learned about a few wild edible plants, but mostly ones that were very common and had no dangerous look-alikes. Grandfather had been very careful with these few plants, pointing them out and warning us of dangers. It was completely different from the other things he taught.

When he came into camp, he sat down and began talking to us about the birds, the weather, and the swamp. Never did he give any clue as to what he was about to teach nor did he even indicate that he wanted to teach us anything. He made mention once to our food and asked us what we would do if we had no food. He got up and left camp, stopping only once to bend over and pick something up, popping it into his mouth. Rick and I paid careful attention to where he had stooped, spying a small patch of greenery. When he was well out of sight, we ran to the patch but were careful not to enter it.

We meticulously retraced his steps, marked the place where he bent over, then spent a good deal of time trying to pinpoint what plant he had eaten. Despite the fact that all the plants were the same type, we took no chances, for it could have been a far different plant growing within the confines of these plant people. We finally spotted the place where the leaf was pulled from the plant. We were certain that it wasn't removed by an animal because of the distinctive tear in the stem instead of a sharp bite. We also searched the ground for prints of other animals to make sure the leaf was not torn loose by a footstep.

Satisfied that this was the plant from which Grandfather had eaten the leaf, we carefully dug up the plant, put it into an old cup, and brought it back to camp for further study. We first looked the plant up in our field guide and found out that it was called wintergreen. We read everything about it, even drew it into our notebooks. We inspected it very carefully so that we would know it in the future. Once our thorough inspection was over, we returned it to its home, watered it, and inspected the other members of its tribe. We found some berries, broke them open, and looked at the seeds. We tore off a leaf, scraped it and took a deep sniff of its fragrance. We were delighted about the way it smelled, making our mouth water. We knew enough, however, not to taste it without asking Grandfather.

We spent the night in the camp area, discussing the new plant, and otherwise goading each other into trying the plant. This constant coaxing and bickering followed us into the next day, but neither of us would budge. We knew the rules and in no way were we going to take a chance in breaking them. We sat by the plants one last time before going home, offering them a little tobacco for what they had taught us. When we got up, we were startled to see Grandfather standing just a few feet from us. Without hesitation, we told him what we had experienced and we wanted to know more about the plant. He only nodded and said that he had been watching us since yesterday and approved of our meticulous effort. He was also delighted that we did not try the plant without asking.

We argued with him about not trying the plant, since we had seen him obviously eat it. He simply said that if he had been taking the plant for some strong medication, then we would have taken the same medication. That could have caused us serious illness. He then asked us if we ever watched the deer or squirrel eat the very poisonous mushrooms with no effect to themselves. Should we risk our lives by eating things that other animals or people eat? We argued with him about the way he had led us to the plant and how he should have stayed and finished his lesson. He told us that we learned far more about the plant by ourselves than we would have if he had pointed it out to us.

Yes, we did eventually learn that the plant was edible, but we learned so much more in the process. We had practiced our tracking, our identification skills, and had studied the plant thoroughly. We also learned patience and to intimately recognize the plant from that day forward. We also learned to discipline ourselves against each other's goading to break the rules. Truly the plant taught us to make our own decisions for ourselves, not because of peer pressure. This little plant and its overall lesson is probably one of the factors involved in keeping me away from drugs and such, even though I was a child of the sixties.

Grandfather led us to the realms of tasting the plant. He asked us to take a new, succulent leaf from the uppermost part, tear off a piece, and place it in our mouths. The flavor seemed to grow more intense as we waited until it filled the whole mouth. It was delicious, but he warned us that the plant was also a powerful medicine and that we should not eat too much. One or two leaves as a trailside nibble was all we should ingest. We came back the next day to savor the berries in the same way, and throughout the rest of the summer and into the fall, we began to know the little plant quite well.

Months later we were on a winter hike with Grandfather. Snow had covered the ground completely and it had been bitter cold for months. We had walked a long way and sat down for a much-needed rest. As Rick and I sat, we watched Grandfather wandering about the immediate landscape looking at the trees and their reference to the ground. It was as if he were looking for a buried treasure. Finally he knelt down, brushed some snow away, picked something up, and ate it. We rushed over to see what this marvelous snow plant might be, for both of us had seen its green. To our amazement it was a little wintergreen, looking as fresh and delicious as the day we had learned about it in the summer.

Grandfather commented that not everything sleeps in the winter, and that certain plants and animals that look frail and weak can actually take more than the stronger plants. Grandfather told us that the little plant gained its power from the Earth. By growing close to the Mothering power, it was protected by the Earth, which kept it warm so it would live even in the winter. He commented that we should learn to do the same.

Food   We used to collect wintergreen leaves for tea anytime of the year. We knew that this plant brother had powerful medicinal properties, so we used it sparingly. Using only a few leaves to a cup of boiling water, we would brew a delicious tea that was both refreshing in the summer and warming in the winter. We would also use the new leaves as a trailside nibble, a component of salads, or a fresh seasoning for cooking. The berries are also quite refreshing and a good trailside nibble when you are on the go. The berries can be found sometimes through the winter into the next spring. They also make a great addition to fry bread, ash cakes, and even pancakes. I find that the crushed berries, mixed with a few leaves, and steeped in hot water for ten minutes make a great hot or cold tea. Make sure that you filter out the tea before drinking.

Medicinal   My first experience with the medicinal properties of wintergreen came as a result of an intense headache. I had been studying for a biology exam in high school, and I had to keep up my grade average, not only because I loved the subject but because Rick was in my class and we had a mild competition going. That meant I had to study every possible moment of the day and well into the night. This intense study schedule went on for a week until we took the exam on Friday. The comedown was intense, not only because the exam was over and we did well, but also because it was the start of a long weekend camping trip. We were so excited about this trip, that with the ups and down, we both got violent headaches.

At first our headaches weren't bad, but as we walked toward Grandfather's camp, we became debilitated with pain. It was supposed to be one of our favorite campouts of the year which we called clam camp. We were to hike well into the night and camp on the edge of Barnegat Bay, where we would clam all weekend and study the vast variety of birdlife. Neither of us would give into the pain, but after a few miles of walking, we really wanted to give up. Grandfather had been watching our pain increase for several hours. When we finally stopped for a rest at mid-journey, he went out and picked some fresh wintergreen leaves from an old plant to use as medication for our headaches.

Despite the pain, we were curious as to how the wintergreen leaves that we used as tea could have any effect on our pain. After all, we had noticed no difference during the times we drank the wintergreen as tea. Grandfather explained that we only used a few leaves for our teas, which we boiled. He was going to use larger leaves and more of them, which he would steep. He took a large palmful of leaves and steeped them in a cup of hot water for over half an hour. We drank a little at a time until we finished the cup. Within an hour, our headaches were gone and we went on to complete the campout. Many years later, I learned that the oils found in the wintergreen leaf contain the chemical, methyl salicylate, which is a close relative of aspirin.

A strong tea of wintergreen also makes a good mouthwash for sore throats, cold sores, and gum ailments. A stronger tea can be brewed as a skin wash for skin problems and irritations. The leaves can also be used in poultice form, but repeated use of the poultice may cause skin irritation. I make a balm from the crushed leaves steeped in hot tallow, then cooled. I find it great for mild burns one may suffer around a campfire. Some old-timers also use wintergreen tea as a pain medication in another form. They breathe in the steam vapors produced by boiling the leaves vigorously.

Wood Sorrel (*Oxalis spp.*)

Description   Wood sorrel loves cool, moist woods. Some of the species prefer open woods and field edges. It is a low, woodland flower, very delicate in appearance and to the touch. The leaves are cloverlike with three heart-shaped leaflets that most times fold along a central crease. The leaves have a sour taste. The flowers are pink, red, or yellow, and flower in late spring to early summer. Wood sorrel is found from Maine and the New England states into Canada, ranging south and east from Pennsylvania to Minnesota near the Great Lakes. It can also be found along the Appalachian Mountains to North Carolina and Tennessee.

Personality   Wood sorrel has long been one of my favorite trailside nibbles and one of the most powerful plant teachers I have ever known. Wood sorrel is not a particularly strong medicine, nor is it a totally flawless food. In fact, it is rather mediocre in most respects. What the wood sorrel had shown me was of the utmost importance, especially in my development as an herbalist. It taught me the final lessons in the inner awareness of communication. It was the real teacher in Grandfather's final lesson, the last thing he taught me before he left.

Wood sorrel did not grow extensively in our area of the Pines, and I was not too familiar with the plant. I did know that it was edible and whenever I found it I would nibble on some. It was not high on my list of wild edible plants, not because it wasn't delicious, but because it was not available in large quantities for survival purposes. Compared to the other plants I used on a daily basis, I knew relatively little about wood sorrel. No book at the time seemed to carry much information about it, either.

One of the things Rick and I used to do was to help Grandfather with his herbal collecting, and we would accompany him whenever he visited a patient. At these times, he would have us help him prepare remedies or collect some fresh herbs if needed. It was during one of these visits to an old cranberry farmer that wood sorrel taught me its profound lesson in communication, thus opening up the door to a greater spiritual understanding of the deeper realms of the natural world. It taught a communication so profound that I cannot deny its wisdom.

Grandfather needed yarrow to treat this old cranberry farmer's mild digestive problem. He could not use any of the more powerful herbs because the farmer suffered from an ulcer and a strong medication would do more harm than good. He was very specific about the type of herb he wanted, what stage of development it was in, what part to take, and where it grew. When Grandfather wanted a particular plant, we knew that we had better get that exact plant and plant part because it was critical to the well-being of the patient.

Rick and I set out to collect the yarrow, which we knew to be rare in this area, and at this time of year it was going to be next to impossible to find one in the exact stage of growth that Grandfather needed. I don't know whether he planned this lesson or it just happened, but it forever changed my life and my sense of reality. Rick and I searched for hours, at best finding only a handful of the yarrow that he wanted, and they were well past the stage he desperately needed. The sun was setting and we had been gone for over half a day, so Rick decided to go back to Grandfather with what he had. I would stay behind and look some more, and then meet him there by dark.

As I sat on an old tree stump feeling sorry for myself and watching the sunset, a little plant by my feet caught my eye. Immediately I identified it as a wood sorrel, but a deeper urge nagged at me to pick it and bring it back to Grandfather. All the logic and past training screamed at me not to take it for it was not what he needed. The inner voice was stronger, however, so I gathered up a good handful of the herb and headed back to Grandfather. I handed Grandfather the herb and told him that these would work better than the herb that he had originally asked for. He smiled and was a bit taken back by the confidence I showed about the herb.

Inquisitively he asked, "How do you know?"

I answered, "I know deep inside and it feels good for this type of ailment."

Rick was sure that I was going to get admonished for my stupidity, but Grandfather only smiled and began to prepare the wood sorrel for the remedy. I was delighted, not only because I had pleased Grandfather, but because I definitely knew without a doubt that this herb was good for that ailment. Later we sat on the front porch of the farmer's home talking. Grandfather was pleased that I had heard the voices of the plant and knew that the plant could be used for that healing. He taught me to nurture that feeling and never allow my logic to stand in the way of such a profound inner feeling. He was delighted that I took that chance and stood my ground, even when he questioned me. He then went on to teach me about unwavering faith. Simply stated, if you need a plant in a particular growth cycle, it or at least a good substitute will be there.

We walked a few yards from the little farmhouse, and there at Grandfather's feet was the plant that Grandfather had originally asked for. To our amazement, it was in the exact stage of growth that he needed. He spoke of allowing our inner voices to lead us right to the plant that we needed, and how we should follow this voice at all times no matter what our logic dictates. He said that our logic had told us that the original plants he needed did not grow readily in this area of the Pines and even if we found any, they would not be in the proper stage of growth because it was too late in the season. By listening to our logic, we had effectively blinded ourselves to all possibilities and to ever seeing the plant we needed. That kind of prejudice, born from the lack of faith, is another form of blindness.

We saw the power of Grandfather's unwavering faith and a great lesson in following the inner voice the last winter we were together. Grandfather was treating a patient of his who was dying of cancer. The medical world had given up and told the old woman that she had only a few months to live. In desperation, even though she did not believe in the superstition of ancient herbology, she summoned Grandfather as a last resort. She was emaciated and looked full of pain; her desperation had made her bitter. Grandfather had to prepare one of his most secret remedies but needed a fresh green plant as a catalyst in order for the medication to work. Both Rick and I knew that it was impossible to find the plant in this section of the Pine Barrens, and even if he did, it was the dead of winter and that plant would be nothing more than a withered skeleton.

We followed Grandfather out into the snowy night. The wind was bitterly cold and merciless. All the fields were covered with a thick blanket of snow, and we knew that there was no way we could complete the medication. But we trusted Grandfather almost as if he were some mystical deity, his every move teaching us something, so we stayed close and followed him no matter how much our logic told us that it wouldn't work. He seemed to drift randomly for a while, not heading in any particular direction. Stopping frequently in an attitude of prayer and worship, he would rest. It was if he were listening to a voice we could not hear. He was eventually led to the edge of a small cedar swamp, where the brush hit the smaller cedars and sourgums.

He bent down on his hands and knees to pray over a little mound of snow before him. Reverently, he got up and began to walk back to the house. We knew that he had failed, so we began to walk after him. He turned to us and asked us why we were following him and not collecting the plant. We sheepishly stated that we didn't see any plant and would not know where to dig. He smiled confidently and said, "Dig where I prayed, and bring back only the flowers and the tiny new leaves."

We were shocked into immobility. After a long while we walked back to the area, knowing that there could never be a plant under all that snow, especially a flowering plant that only lives once through the warmer months of the summer.

Holding the torchlight and lightly brushing the snow from the mound, we began to dig down. We knew there would be no plant but we respected Grandfather enough to try. There in the shelter of a fallen log shone the bright flower of a wood sorrel. Its leaves and flower looked as fresh as if it were spring, and its beauty sparkled in the torchlight like no other flower we'd ever seen. Both Rick and I cried, not only for finding the flower, but for our failure in absolute faith. To us it was nothing short of a miracle. The old woman with cancer did not die of it. Six months after the time she was supposed to die they could find no trace of cancer. Call it spontaneous regeneration or call it an herbal miracle, regardless, she lived for many more years, a rich and healthy life. Since then I've witnessed countless miracles and I have since realized that the greatest gift from the wood sorrel has been the gift of faith.

Food Wood sorrel is a plant that comes with a warning. Essentially, it teaches us the wisdom of moderation. Excess consumption of wood sorrel over a period of time inhibits the body's ability to absorb calcium. However, this should not preclude the use of sorrel as a good wild, edible plant. I use wood sorrel as a trailside nibble, eating the new succulent green leaves. They have a delicious but sour taste that is quite refreshing on hot, summer days. The new green leaves can also be added fresh to salads as a type of spice. Once you familiarize yourself with the taste of wood sorrel, you can use it as a seasoning in so many other dishes.

To make a refreshing drink, steep the leaves in hot water for ten minutes. I suggest a palmful of leaves to a pint of water. Chill, sweeten to taste, and drink like iced tea. Providing the tea isn't boiled, it retains its very rich content of vitamin C. Grandfather would mix one-half wood sorrel tea and one-half herbal tea to produce a very fine hot tea. I have also found hot wood sorrel tea quite delicious, but many people prefer it cold.

Medicinal Wood sorrel is a mild medicinal plant. The chilled tea made from wood sorrel leaves has a tremendous soothing effect on the digestive system. It can be used for the relief of heartburn, cramps, and other digestive disorders. A strong tea can be used as a skin wash for most skin maladies, except deep wounds. This strong tea can also be used as a mouthwash. The herb works best when fresh. Wood sorrel contains oxalic acid which, used excessively, can cause internal irritation that can result in bleeding and diarrhea. Generally, wood sorrel should be used sparingly and with great caution. Wood sorrel's greatest medicinal value is in its catalytic properties.

Yarrow (*Achillea millefolium*)

Description   Yarrow is a beautiful plant with flat-topped clusters of flowers. Each flower contains five petallike rays. The leaves are narrow, lacy, fernlike, and very aromatic. At first glance, they seem to have a woolly appearance. It loves old fields, waste grounds, and sunny places. Yarrow is found throughout the United States.

Personality   The darkness and heat of the sweat lodge cut out all distractions of the outside world. There we sat, symbolically in Earth Mother's womb, waiting for the purification of the steam and the healing powers of the Earth to enter us. This was the holy place of prayer, a symbol of rebirth and a close union to the Creator. There in the darkness there was total concentration on the words, prayers, and songs to the Creator. There we could think deeply, unobstructed by any influence. The sweat lodge is sacred, like a temple within the temple of the universe.

It was in this lodge by the river where we would meet with Grandfather for the spiritual teachings, the purification, the prayers, and to look deeply into ourselves and others. It engendered the reality of brotherhood and brought to light the inner connection and love of true brotherhood. So many times I watched Grandfather enter a sweat lodge to help him focus on knowing one of his patients better. I would also witness him take patients in with him so that his full concentration would be on that person, and he could become a hollow vessel of the Creator and the Earth. There he would administer herbs or put healing herbs directly on the rocks to reach their full power. The lodge was not only a place of prayer and spiritual communion but also a place of healing and purification.

Yarrow was a powerful healer and teacher in the sweat lodge. Grandfather considered it one of the most powerful, especially when used in the magic of the sweat lodge. Its gathering had to be precise, the prayers full of meaning, and the preparation and use of the herb utterly perfect. The teachings of the sweat lodge were a profound statement in purity. Every part of the lodge, from the building of it to the final steam, had to be precise. Each entity of the lodge had to have the proper prayers and be gathered in a prescribed way. Each movement and part was a philosophy unto itself. To light a sweat lodge fire by any other means than a bow drill or hand drill was considered a sacrilege. If the essence of the building of the sacred flame was removed or done artificially then a huge part of the philosophy was missing. The lodge then became powerless.

216

Yarrow has always been bound in mystery, whether used in or out of the sweat lodge. Its power to me is utterly sacred and I will remember to this day the way I learned of its use and power. In the various fields we passed through as children, there would always be a group of the yarrow people there to stimulate our curiosity. Yarrow is one of the most mystical plants in appearance that I know. Its leaves are a source of beautiful fascination and its flowers feed the spirit with their lacy tapestries. The first time I knelt down by one of these little plants, Grandfather came over and sat by me. He waited for a long moment, studying my reaction to the plant. I suspect that he was looking at the way the plant affected me on a spiritual level. Finally he said, "This is a sacred plant which you will someday learn. Treat it so."

From that day on Rick and I had the highest respect for yarrow. It wasn't something understood but rather something from deep inside, innate and uncultured but still a very powerful awareness. It was a feeling of being in the presence of the unseen and eternal. It served as our first real lesson in the spiritual presence of an inner voice, an inner awareness and communication. The plant enraptured us and we held it in utter awe every time we gazed upon it, yet on the physical plane we knew nothing of it whatsoever. To us it was as mystically powerful as the sweat lodge that we were just beginning to understand. The plant brought out something in us from deep inside, a type of yearning as if something were trying to talk to us but we could not yet hear.

It was years later that Grandfather finally allowed us to touch a yarrow plant. We had to understand more about it and be closer to Creation before he would allow us to understand the sensuality of its touch. As we sat by a particular patch of yarrow people one day, Grandfather offered the largest plant a gift of tobacco and a prayer. He then carefully broke off a lacy leaf found from another plant. Rubbing it gently between his fingers, he lifted it to his nose and inhaled deeply. His expression was nothing less than total rapture. He passed it to us and motioned for us to do the same. We were beyond delight, almost intoxicated by the fragrance. Nothing in the natural world smelled so fine, so powerful, and so pure. It felt as if we had savored the essence of a spirit, not a plant.

Again, years passed before we learned anything more about yarrow. It was in the dark confines of a sweat lodge, gazing into the hot rocks, which were glowing a transparent red-orange. We sat for a long time in silent reverence, feeling the essence of the dry heat and awaiting the cleansing steam to begin. Our minds drifted to the powers beyond simple sight and sound, to a realm that we could feel even though it was beyond our understanding. Then the prayer from Grandfather began and the herb was dropped on the hot rocks. The aroma had a mysterious power that we could not understand. It was not like any other sacred herb but had a fragrance all its own. The fragrance seemed to reach deep inside, telling us instantly that Grandfather had used yarrow in this lodge for the sacred herb.

The scent of the yarrow seemed to stay with us through the constant washing waves of steam. Our minds drifted through endless chasms, quieting at times as our spirits began to soar free. Hours went by, and then a cup was passed between us. We tasted the bitter brew and the scent told us that it was made of yarrow. Grandfather poured the remainder of the tea onto the rocks and the room filled with a thick scent. Our bodies began to sweat profusely as they never had before in any lodge. Our relaxation was profound and our meditation deep. The scent of the yarrow was always with us and growing more powerful with each wave of steam. It was as if we were enveloped in the steamy spirit of the plant, its essence so utterly strong that we could almost touch it.

From this first baptism in the steam of yarrow tea, my respect for the plant has grown tremendously. I hold it in absolute awe and consider it one of the most sacred of plants to this day. I have seen Grandfather use the plant to stop bleeding, reduce a violent fever, and wash wounds. I've seen the power of yarrow heal where other remedies, even modern medications, have failed miserably. Yarrow is powerful by itself and is also a prime ingredient in some of the most potent herbal medications. It is because of the sacredness with which I hold the yarrow plant that I cannot convey to the readers all of its uses.

The first real medicinal use of the yarrow that I ever witnessed was during a severe winter storm. One of Grandfather's patients had a severe fever that would not come down under conventional means. Aspirin could barely touch it and cold baths only worked temporarily. Grandfather was called in because the patient was getting worse and the doctor hadn't shown up yet. Apparently, the storm had kept the town at a standstill. Grandfather, using yarrow and another herb, brewed a tea and had his patient drink it slowly over the course of a few hours. The fever came down to a reasonable level within fifteen minutes and was near normal within an hour.

Grandfather used yarrow also as a skin wash but he warned that the prolonged exposure to yarrow wash makes the skin sensitive to sunlight. That is why we only used it rarely in the sweat lodge and then only at night, followed by a vigorous bath. Yarrow as a skin wash is very powerful and can reduce skin maladies and irritations remarkably fast. I have seen Grandfather also stop nose bleeds and internal bleeding with a strong tea of yarrow mixed with other herbs as catalysts. Generally, yarrow should be considered as one of the most powerful herbs and is best left alone.

Food The dried leaves of yarrow brewed in hot water for ten to fifteen minutes make an excellent and healthful tea. It was so sacred to Grandfather that he rarely drank it as a tea and only after he felt that he was in need of a tonic to preserve good health. Caution should be used, however, because yarrow tea does induce sweating.

Medicinal When Grandfather gave us yarrow tea to drink in the sweat lodge, he had a dual purpose in mind. First he was using the tea as a health drink since we were in the heart of the flu season. Secondly, he wanted to produce a profuse sweating during the time we were in the lodge, and the tea would induce such a sweat. Grandfather would use the tea also in alleviating fever but it was best mixed with an aspirin-bearing plant such as wintergreen. The wintergreen and yarrow tea mixture was one of the better cold tonics and one of the best for bringing down a fever. The dosage of tea should fit the patient. Use a palmful of dried herb to one cup of water. Use one cup a day for only two days, then discontinue use. This is the average dosage for most patients but sometimes a stronger tea is needed.

A good use of yarrow tea is to use it as a skin wash for all types of infections and irritations. The only drawback is that the repeated use causes sensitivity to sunlight so it must be used infrequently. I use yarrow tea as a skin wash for bad infections or irritations when all else fails. For tenacious boils and pimples, I use the fresh, crushed yarrow leaves applied directly to the infected area. Keep bandaged in sunlight. It also seems to help draw out the inflammation. Yarrow can also be used to effectively stop or slow internal bleeding, but the procedure and medication mixtures are too extensive and a bit dangerous to be covered in this book.

Yarrow varies in taste, and I know that it varies in potency depending on where it grows and what stage of growth it is in. The strongest time for collecting yarrow is just before the flowers are produced, using only the new succulent leaves. It is also good to collect the yarrow just before a rain and from areas where the soil is rich. Pick yarrow plants that are not exposed to the sun all day long, but not ones that are extensively shaded. Dry yarrow leaves slowly in a cool dark place and store in a glass or earthenware container. It is best not to keep the container tightly sealed. Store the container in a cool and dry place out of direct sunlight.

Yucca (*Yucca filamentosa*)

Description Yucca is a lover of sandy woods, old fields, and sandy waste areas. It has long swordlike leaves that terminate in a sharp point. This evergreen plant flowers from late spring to midsummer. Its flowers have six petals, appearing waxy white. It grows long stalks in large terminal clusters. Yucca is found in the southwestern United States and along the coastal plains of Georgia, north into New Jersey. This plant is often cultivated and may be established farther north.

Personality Grandfather was raised in the southwestern United States and in Mexico for much of his early life. He then began to wander this country extensively, eventually penetrating up into Canada and Alaska, and as far south as Panama. His stories were rich with culture and of the animals and plants of various areas. He was especially fond of the plants found in his homeland. Many of the plants had stories connected with their uses, or songs that went with the collection or preparation of the plant. One plant in particular stands out in my mind, not only because it was one of the first plants I learned, but because it was also a native of Grandfather's homeland. He had so many stories and mysteries surrounding the yucca plant that it seemed endless in its uses.

One of the first uses of yucca we learned was cordage. This is probably one of the first work songs I ever learned, and it stays with me to this day. One of the steps in extracting the cordage fibers from the yucca leaves is to rhythmically pound the leaves with a wooden mallet against a hardwood anvil. It works best when a rhythm is kept up, for the fibers come out even and the work seems to fly. With this repetitive rhythm came a wealth of songs and chants, which Grandfather would sing while working. It was the yucca-fiber work song that we learned first.

The plant itself was a mystery to us. It looked so out of place in the sandy areas of the Pine Barrens, as if it had escaped from the Southwest but it was quite at home in this area. Just like the prickly pear cactus, it belonged here and made life easier. I have found it also in areas where it usually would not be. This is because it is extensively cultivated as a garden plant and sometimes escapes when conditions are right. To a survivalist, the plant has seemingly endless possibilities. To start with, it makes one of the strongest cordages. This cordage is so strong that it will easily pull back a seventy-five-

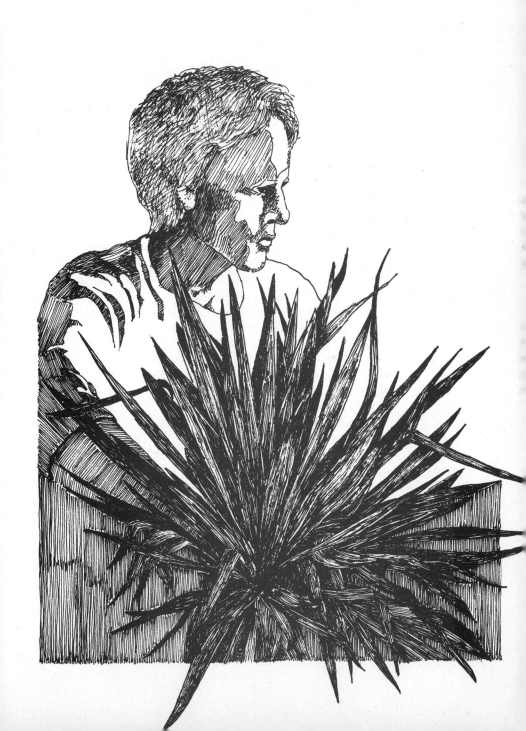

pound bow, using an average diameter bowstring. We also used the leaves to weave baskets and mats, as well as make a number of other strong cordage-based products.

We also learned to dig the roots. These contained sophins that would produce a lather when pounded in water. The soap made from yucca root was very effective in cleaning, though very mild to the skin and hair. In fact, we found that soap made from yucca root would actually make the hair and skin look much healthier. Rick and I would make extra money or barter with the homemade shampoo that we would make from yucca root and a few other herbs. To this day, I sometimes make up shampoo for my students or my family but, beg as they may, I'll never disclose all the herbs used.

The first time I used yucca as a food was on a trip to the estuary area of Long Beach Island. Long Beach Island is a landmass just off the coast of New Jersey that was once a sandbar of some sort. At that time, it was well endowed with houses and other buildings, and it is still a summer resort. The Pine Barrens lay directly to the west, and we could easily walk the bridge to the island to do our clamming and fishing. Though there was plenty to eat in the way of plants, we dare not take any because the dunescape was very fragile and the removal of them would cause an extreme sand shift. This posed a little difficulty in that we would rarely bring any food with us, and we would have to go back to the Pine Barrens after one day.

On one beautiful summer day, we decided to venture onto the island and do some clamming as well as watch the shorebirds. We got so caught up in the wonders of the lower end of the island, which is otherwise deserted, that we forgot to watch the time. We watched the sunset and then built a small shelter into which the three of us could fit. The sleep was profound and beautiful, having been lulled by the rhythm of the waves. However, the next morning we awoke starving with nothing to eat anywhere. We had not fished or clammed the day before so we were also out of meat.

We followed Grandfather to the main part of the island. The houses were quiet and there were no cars out yet. Not even the sun had risen into the sky. Water was also at a premium on that lower part of the island and we were more thirsty than we were hungry. I thought that we were going onto the inhabited part of the island to drink from someone's faucet and buy something to eat at the general store, but Grandfather had other ideas. In the misty dawn, we passed yucca bush after yucca bush, cultivated by the beach people as a garden plant. Grandfather would stop periodically and peel off a flower petal and eat it, and it didn't take us long before we were doing the same. In a short while, our appetites were eased and the dew on the petals gave us plenty of water.

It was funny to watch people's expressions as they gazed at us eating the yucca flowers. To them, we must have looked like a motley group from another planet or a bunch of hermits right out of the woods. We finally headed back to the south end of the island when a local home owner threatened to call the police on us for destroying his plants. All the explaining in the world would not convince him that we were not hurting the plants, so we departed hastily.

This book was written almost entirely in a small house on the same island. Before writing about the yucca plant, I took a trip back to the place where we had first eaten the yucca flowers, hoping to rekindle the feeling I had back then. Lost in thought, I began munching the petals of one particular yucca, probably the same one I had eaten twenty-three years ago. Again, a man came out of the house and began to scream at me to get out of his garden. The first day I had ever eaten the flower lived all over again, except with a different ending. Realizing who I was, he ran back to the house and reappeared with my first book and asked me to autograph it for him. He then ate some yucca petals with me.

As I write my books, either with a co-author or by myself, I like to revisit the places where I originally learned about the plant. Today, it is becoming more and more difficult. Many of the areas where I grew up have now been developed or turned into factories. Other areas are now too close to civilization and the possibility of pollution precludes the eating of plants. Most of the old people that Grandfather loved have been swept away with the flood of houses, and many of the old herbalists are now gone. Just as I showed the gentleman how to eat yucca, which he now cultivates with a vengeance, all of us should teach whomever we can so that this cancerous destruction can stop.

Food   The flower petals of the yucca plant can be eaten raw or added to salads. They have an uncommon taste and are utterly delicious. Yucca does not make an all-round survival food because it has few edible parts. However, there are so many uses of yucca on a utilitarian basis that it becomes a relished survival companion.

Medicinal   The medicinal value of yucca lies in the soap content of the root. Generally the yucca root can be pounded into an effective but mild soap. The soap is great for washing sores, cuts, damaged hair, and for many other skin maladies. I have also found it effective in treating cold sores by diluting it into a mouthwash. A poultice of the root can also be used to drain boils, remove insect stings, and stop the incessant itch of poison ivy. Do not allow it to stay on skin any longer than one-half hour. Wash off thoroughly.

PART THREE

A Plant Story

The plant people are critical to the existence of mankind. Yet every day man destroys that which keeps him alive. We have become a society that kills its grandchildren to feed its children. We have lost our connection to the Earth and can no longer see the umbilical cord that sustains our lives. Man's removal from the Earth has caused an ignorance and complacency, as well as a false sense of security. Because mankind does not feel the effects of his indiscriminate destruction firsthand, he continues butchering the Earth, falsely believing that we will never run out of trees or other living things. Through the doorway of survival, humankind can experience firsthand the importance of plants to his life, and possibly rebuild the reverence and awe for the land that he so desperately lacks.

I do not expect everyone to run out into the wilderness and begin to live a survival existence. We would soon run out of places for people to find seclusion, and most of our life-styles would not permit such a long vacation. If I can impart unto you the essence of a survival situation as I have lived it, then perhaps you can see what an intricate part the plant people play in our lives. By understanding the way plants form such a dynamic reality in a survival situation, one can easily realize the connection between the modern self and the umbilical cord of Earth Mother.

After years of trial and error in perfecting my skills, I can clearly see the awesome link between myself and the Earth. I realize that I am not better than the other entities of Creation, but equal and dependent on them. I understand that without them, my life would soon come to a halt. Without the proper and sacred use of these entities, we could run out of them later on, even in our own lifetime. Coming from a life of survival living, I accept the sacred responsibility of being a caretaker of the Earth, without removing myself to some outside Godlike plane. I am as subject to the laws of Creation as anything else, and as with anything else, I will die if I violate them. The reverence I feel for the awesome responsibility of the ultimate gift—life giving up life so I can live—permeates my every move. I am always thankful for all things given to me. Every act and every move is a sacred experience, for I truly dwell in the temples of God.

As I enter the wilderness and drop my clothing, I am returning to our Earth Mother. I must put trust in my skills and my ability to be one with, and trust that the Earth will fill all my needs. I look caringly for a place to put my shelter. I am looking for a place that is surrounded by small trees and brush that will protect my shelter from the prevailing winds and storms. I am looking for a place that will provide the materials needed to build the shelter and the wood to keep my fires going. The plant people make my cradle and protect me from the storms of existence. Here in this plant cradle I will find the security I need to survive, for all around me are the help and protection of the plant people.

I then begin to build my shelter. Rocks and earth would make a suitable shelter but not without the wood to create the inner fire to keep it warm. Instead, I build a shelter wholly from plants. It is a shelter that needs neither internal fire nor blanket to keep me warm. The old skeletons of branches and sticks become the skeleton of my shelter and make it strong and safe. The debris and litter of the plants in the form of dead leaves, grasses, ferns, mosses, and other old plant material gives me the insulation to keep me warm. It is piled high into a dome, like a huge squirrel nest, which will shed water or wind easily. My inner bed is constructed of piled or woven grasses, made soft and luxurious by the drying effects of the wind's caressing the plants. When my shelter is completed I am cradled in a temple of plants, protected by plants, and wholly kept alive by plants.

As I go about the thirsty job of building my shelter, the plant people will also come to the rescue. Water and food can be had at any time from the succulent assortment of leaves and stems available to me on all landscapes as trailside nibbles. This day I may cut the end of a wild grape vine and take enough water for several days, or I may tap any number of nonsyrup trees for their sap, or depending on place, I may even use a certain cactus for water. Other plants contribute to the making of rivers, streams, and lakes as they hold fast the soils and create natural catches. Earth and water would run wild without the intricate and interlocking root systems of the plants.

I next find the materials I need for my fire. Fire begins and ends with the wisdom of wood. I comb the landscape, seeking out the perfect parts of my bow or hand drill. There I sample all types of dried wood and herbacious stem. I weave together dogbane or velvetleaf fibers to make strong cordage for my fire bow. I collect nut oil, leaf oil, or pine pitch to make the lubricant for my hand hold. I gather dried grasses, roots, and plant fibers to make into my tinder bundle which will be used to cradle, nurture, and feed my tiny coal to flame. Then I collect the various firewoods for my fire. Some woods will give me quick heat and light, some will give me long-lasting

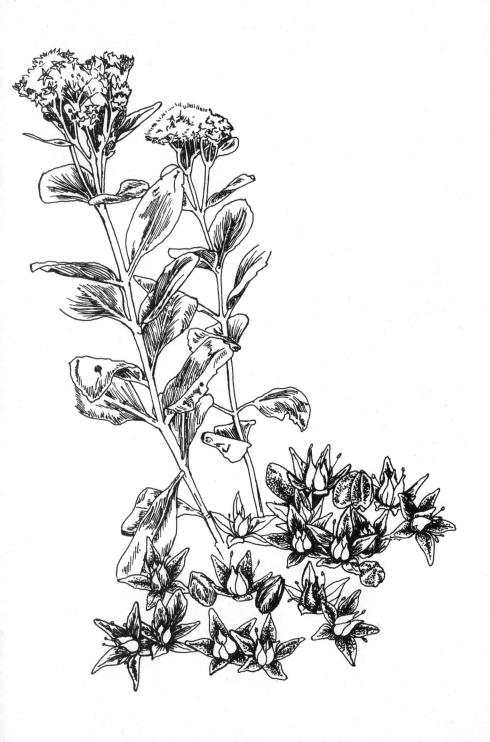

heat and coals, and there are some collected for how quickly or intensely they burn, or how little smoke they give off. My fire is made from the friction of the bow drill, which creates a tiny coal that is unlocked from the hard sunshine we call wood. As the fire burns, I release back to the sky the sunshine and warmth that has been stored for centuries.

The fire from the wood keeps me warm, gives me light, cooks my food, and helps me make the other tools necessary for survival. I use the coals of this sunshine to burn the deep hollows in wood that will become my bowls, and I use the fire to cut and shape other wood. The fire will also harden the tip of a throwing spear, or bake my clay pots that have been shaped by wooden spatulas and gouges. The fire is a gift of sunshine, held only by the plant people. For years it has been a source of magic, fuel for introspection, and a sacred purifier. I often wonder what locks our hypnotic gaze to a campfire: Is it the reverence for the gift of wood, or is it the magic that has spellbound mankind since the dawn of time? Fire has been instrumental in our evolution, and has come to us as a sacred gift from the plants.

After my camp is secure with a good shelter, bedding, water, and fire, the plant people also enable me to hunt and gather. I gather from the landscape a fire-killed ash, hickory, ironwood, or yew, then carve it into a bow. The shaping is done with stone tools held fast by wooden handles. The bow is steamed then bent into a beautiful recurve, using smooth round log halves as a form and wooden clamp pegs to hold in place. My arrows are collected also, usually from small fire-killed saplings that have grown very straight. These are also formed and shaped by the steam from the fire or by the stone or bone tools held fast by wooden handles. In times of lack, pine needles or plant fiber can be used as arrow fletching, bound fast to the shaft by cordage when sinew is unavailable. When there is no stone or bone to make arrow points, the wood of the very shaft or other hardwood points can be fire-hardened into serviceable tips.

It is a source of wonder how mankind has to take a life to take a life. The gifts are never ending and very profound. Here man must remove the life of the tree from the landscape, then shape it into a tool which in reality is an extension of self, a specialized appendage. Here man uses that bow and arrow, harmless trees at one time, for a killing tool. Here the power of the tree and sapling, sunshine, Earth, and water are transformed into the death of an animal, which further becomes another extension of man. Without that magical transformation of plant into the tools of man, man would not survive. To humankind who live close to the Earth, the plants are always mystical, magical, and full of wisdom.

I then select small saplings from the landscape and produce my traps. Configurations of sticks form triggers for deadfalls and snares, and the cordage for the snares is from plants, too. Most of my traps will then be baited by plants, and it is the juice from aromatic plants that camouflage my scent around the trap sight. Saplings are also made into fish spears and fish traps as my use of plants reaches into lakes and streams. From plant fiber I weave intricate patterns of nets, and small balls of wood will keep these nets afloat. The fish that I catch are dried on wooden racks or mats, and sometimes even cooked on wooden slats. The catch is stored in baskets woven of plant fiber, cordage, or slats hammered from wood.

Most of my meat and larder is stored in these baskets and my camp is made more comfortable as I accumulate other products made from plants. Once I have taken care of all of my needs, I then take care of my wants. I begin to make soft luxurious blankets and outer-garments from pounded cedar fiber. Workbenches are made from fallen logs. Backrests are manufactured by stringing saplings together side by side, so that my campfire seat is as comfortable as a lounge chair. To light the camp area, torches are made out of cattail, mullein, or teasel. Various hardwoods are collected to produce the exact smoke I needed to smoke my food or finish my buckskin clothing. That same smoke is used as a camouflager of scent and a fumigant of shelter areas. The charred wood becomes a means to darken and camouflage my skin.

The necessities and comforts that the plants fulfill go on and on. I use the pounded bark of birch for toothpaste and the inner part of a cattail stalk as a toothbrush, once the seeds are removed. I use meadowsweet and so many other plants as soaps to clean body, hair, and wound. Other plants, hung strategically in my shelter, keep out insects while the burning of other plants act as insecticides. So many other plants make dyes for my clothing, glues, oils, greases, cordages, tinctures, medications, and food. Each stage in the development of my camp utilizes more and more plants. If care is not taken in the harvesting of these plants, then I will find myself living on a desert. Very much like the desert that will one day overtake this country if man does not strike a balance between himself and the land.

Plants can go on to help me build bigger shelters. A long-term, easy-living shelter that I call the earth shelter is made up of bark stripped from dead trees. These shelters can accommodate quite a few people and are very comfortable. These more permanent shelters teach mankind a dynamic balanced attitude toward the landscape. Man can no longer move and allow the land to replenish itself as his ancestors did. He must learn to care for it as he uses it so that it is always rich and productive for all generations. This takes great wisdom and unselfish foresight.

We can also use the plant people to build canoes of bark or dugouts of tree trunks, and we can use wooden paddles or woven sails to propel them. There is no limit to the utilitarian gifts that the plant people give to us in a survival situation.

My medical supplies are as intricate and diverse as the plant people that surround me. I use spagnum moss or the inner barks of certain trees for bandages. Not only do they keep the wound clean, but they also guard against infection with their astringent properties. For internal problems, I can choose from hundreds of different plants. Some can be used to stop diarrhea, some for constipation, some for cramps, poor digestion, heartburn, upset stomach, ulcer, internal bleeding, and as an overall tonic for good health. Other plants can be used as pain-killers for specific and nonspecific pain. Some are especially good for headaches, some relieve joint pain, some relieve muscle pain, and some will soothe all pain. Some plants reduce fever, congestion, and clogged sinuses, and relieve cold or flu symptoms. And many can be used as skin washes for any skin malady. I believe there is not a disease on Earth that there is not a plant to cure it.

Mixtures of plants in my plant pharmacy are even more intricate and involved. Where one specific plant will not work on an ailment, a combination of two or more will get the job done. The mixtures and dosages are as precise as the seasons and each plant varies in strength, depending on its growth cycle and soil or weather conditions. The herbology science is an exacting one, passed down from generation to generation through apprenticeship and vast time spent in the field. These medicines are so important to the survivalist and wanderer who can't get back to civilization to get help and must fend for themselves.

My food is also of great variety and tastes. I make flours and grains for breads and cereals from acorns, reed and cattail roots, tubers, stems, and seeds of all sorts. My breads are more delicious and healthful than those found in any health-food bakery. I dine also on fresh greens, roots, stems, leaves, seeds, nuts, berries, grains, tubers, and flowers. All come with a variety of recipes and seasonings to make tasty dishes that rival anything found at home or in a restaurant. All are fresh and without preservatives, pure and natural food at its finest. Even though I will cultivate some foods and medicinals, there is nothing artificial or harmful used. I can blend my gardens right into the landscape so that the trained observer will not even know that they are there.

Most of all, I share my plants with all the entities of Creation. When I cultivate gardens or take care of the landscapes, it is not only done for myself but for the thousands of other things that feed on the plants. Even if I will never visit an area again, I always leave it well cared for or improved for the next survivalist or those creatures that make their homes there. I also experiment with various plants and how they grow in certain cultivated survival conditions. Some of the best plants I have cultivated for all-around survival food are cattails and amaranths. I believe that some day they will be found growing as a cultivated crop throughout the country. Both will prove far superior to the cultivated crops that we grow now.

I am also a firm believer that the cures for some of man's most dreaded diseases will come from the plant people. These cures can be found right now if only science will listen to the power of the old herbalists and healers. I have seen the natural herbs help cure things that have not responded to science, medicine, or artificial drugs. Even though I believe in the great job that science and medicine is doing, I still think that mankind has far to go. Prejudice is keeping modern man away from many of the cures and medicines that are part of a tradition, thus stifling his advance because of his own arrogance. I have a saying with my students: When all else fails, come and see me. I have seen the things the herbs can do and I know that it is not mere superstition. Superstition does not produce results.

No matter how far man's feet are removed from the soil, he is still connected to the Earth and especially to the plants. The problem is that modern society is blocked from seeing the Earth by the supermarkets and the pharmacies. Mankind does not see the wheat or corn grow, or the cattle being slaughtered, or the countless plants going into his food, medications, cosmetics, and so many of the other things that he uses daily. Some people will even read this book and fail to see the trees that once grew strong and tall, slaughtered for this paper. No matter how far we are removed or how blinded to the connection of Earth we are, we cannot escape it, nor can we ignore it and all its problems. The saving of the Earth is not a problem that we can ignore and hope it will go away. We cannot rely on others to bear the burden either, for all too many have run away and hid in the hills from this responsibility.

The saving of the Earth, the plant and animal people, the air, the waters, and the old ways are important to our survival. We have got to get our head out of the sand and look deeper than the super-markets. We have to realize that everything is interconnected and affects everything else. The devastation of a small patch of natural land in a crowded town is as destructive as the selling of farmland for housing or the butchering of virgin timber for parking lots. We can't allow ourselves to become complacent in our beliefs that some pieces of land do not matter. We have to stop killing our grandchildren to feed our children and our greed.

Simply stated, this whole society is based on a single blade of grass. All our meat and grains come from the grasses and the grasses hold our soils. When that one blade of grass is finally destroyed, it will tip the balance of the Earth toward total destruction. But which blade of grass is it? Could it be the one that is dying from acid rain now? Or the one about to be plowed under to make a freeway, a parking lot, a shopping center, a housing project? Or could it be the one about to be killed by a chemical dump? When will the balance be tipped? When man's greed finally destroys the Earth and produces water lines where water is sold for more than gas, where food is scarce, and where life is no longer tolerable on this planet. That's when the children of the Earth will run to the mountains and ask the rocks to fall on them. That is when Armageddon will come. When the skies bleed the very fire of the holocaust, that is when we will know the blade of grass has fallen.

Now! Out to the Field

When I first sat down to write this book, I had set my goals far too high. I had wanted to cover the uses of more than one hundred plant species, but I fell far short of my goal. So much information had to be cut from each plant, leaving only the raw use without the thousands of other uses. For example, as you read the section on yarrow, you must realize that those final pages were cut down from over one hundred pages of information. I have left out, in many cases, some utilitarian uses, the dyes, the tools, many of the more intricate medicinal uses, the uses as catalysts, and so many of the other edible parts. It has become painfully apparent that this guide will only be the beginning of what should be a long series of books, hopefully containing over fifteen hundred plant species found in the United States.

The reason for the format of the book is simple. I was tired of seeing so many plant books on the market today that were too technical and boring. Upon finishing one of these books, a student hardly knows the plant at all, and the information is soon forgotten. I believe that all plants have unique spirits and that each has a marvelous story. I wanted to incorporate these stories into my text to add form and dimension to each plant so that the student could know them intimately as I do. My ambition is to make the study of plants exciting and interesting to the beginner as well as the seasoned herbalist.

The medicinal values of plants stated in this book are not hearsay. Instead, they have been passed along to me from the ancients or come from my own experience with them. I do not dwell on half-truths and had tested each plant many times before they became the truths of this book. I do not teach from hearsay or about a plant that I have only used a few times. I teach only those plants that have proved their value to me and so many others with reproducible results. In all cases, I have tried to be cautious with the uses of the plants, making sure the dosages were average and effective on most people. Remember, some of you could be allergic to plants, so use them sparingly at first.

A good way to test a known wild edible plant is to identify it correctly, using a good field guide such as *Peterson's Field Guide to Edible Wild Plants* or the *Field Guide to the Wildflowers*. Once positively identified, sample a small portion of the plant and wait a few hours. If there are no side effects, try a little more, then a little more until you are sure that you have no allergy or adverse reaction to the plant. Always positively identify the plant as if your life depended on it, because in essence it does. Always use extreme conservation and caution in gathering plants. Sloppiness will lead to the gathering of plants of other species that could be poisonous, inadvertently mixed in with the ones you would eat. Always check through each plant bunch to insure no unwanted plants or diseased plants have been collected mistakenly. Caution should be a primary rule.

Practice the wild edible plants every day. You can't know a plant until you have studied it and tried it. The best way to accomplish a dynamic understanding and kinship with plants is to augment your diet at home, using wild edible plants whenever possible. The more you practice and sample, the more you will know. Learning the lists of plants and their pictures does not really teach the plant, and many deadly mistakes can be made. Simply, to touch is to know. To taste is to understand.

I am not prescribing any plants as a medication. The medicinal values of the plants in this book are the plants I have used in survival situations when I could not get to a doctor or pharmacy. They are also used by me for my general health maintenance and have been adopted and proven by so many of my students. I am still in favor of modern medical attention when the situation merits it, and unless you know plants very well, I would not attempt treating yourself or anyone else with medicinal herbs. More damage can be done through ignorance.

Practice is the magic word. The more you practice the better you will become. The ignorance factor is diminished with each quality hour you spend learning the plants firsthand. Though this book can be enjoyed immensely by the proverbial armchair naturalist and makes a relaxing read, it is still written and outlined with the workings of a field guide in mind. People want things all too quickly today, but plants can only be learned and understood slowly, one plant at a time. The study of plants is not undertaken like a study in economics in college where everything is found in a textbook. The workbook to this field guide is located in the best university in the world: nature coupled with your intense interest and experience.

Remember, 90 percent of the individual plant information had to be cut out, otherwise this book would only contain a handful of plants. If you have any questions about the plant people and have exhausted all possible sources, then I suggest that you attend one of my survival, nature, and tracking courses at the Tracker Survival School or write to me at Box 173, Asbury, New Jersey 08802. My only interest is passing on the old ways, the spirit of oneness with Creation, and preserving the ancient teachings before they are lost forever.

Index